SUPERFOODS
ANTI-AGING

NOTE

This publication was written by registered dietitians to provide insights into better eating habits to promote health and wellness. It does not provide a cure for any specific ailment or condition and is not a substitute for the advice and/or treatment given by a licensed physician.

First published in French in 2015 by Les Publications Modus Vivendi Inc.
under the title *Superaliments anti-âge*.
© Elisabeth Cerqueira, Marise Charron and Les Publications Modus Vivendi Inc., 2017

MODUS VIVENDI PUBLISHING INC.

55 Jean-Talon Street West
Montreal, Quebec H2R 2W8
CANADA

modusvivendipublishing.com

Publisher: Marc G. Alain
Editorial director: Isabelle Jodoin
Content and copy editor: Nolwenn Gouezel
English-language editor: Carol Sherman
Translator: Kate Bernard
Proofreader: Sasha Regehr
Graphic designer: Émilie Houle
Food photographer: André Noël (anoelphoto.com)
Food stylist: Gabrielle Dalessandro
Authors' and superfoods photographer: Camille Gyrya (camillegyrya.com)

Additional photography:
Pages 4, 5, 8, 9, 10, 11, 14, 17, 21, 31, 39, 43, 45, 47, 48, 53, 58, 59, 60, 61 and 62: Dreamstime.com
Pages 56, 57, 65, 66 and 208: iStock

ISBN: 978-1-77286-030-6 (PAPERBACK)

ISBN: 978-1-77286-031-3 (PDF)
ISBN: 978-1-77286-032-0 (EPUB)
ISBN: 978-1-77286-033-7 (KINDLE)

Legal deposit – Bibliothèque et Archives nationales du Québec, 2017
Legal deposit – Library and Archives Canada, 2017

Government of Quebec – Tax Credit for Book Publishing – Program administered by SODEC

Funded by the Government of Canada

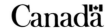

Printed in Canada

SUPERFOODS
ANTI-AGING

Over 50 recipes to slow down the effects of aging

ELISABETH CERQUEIRA AND MARISE CHARRON, RD

With the collaboration of Nolwenn Gouezel

MODUS VIVENDI

CONTENTS

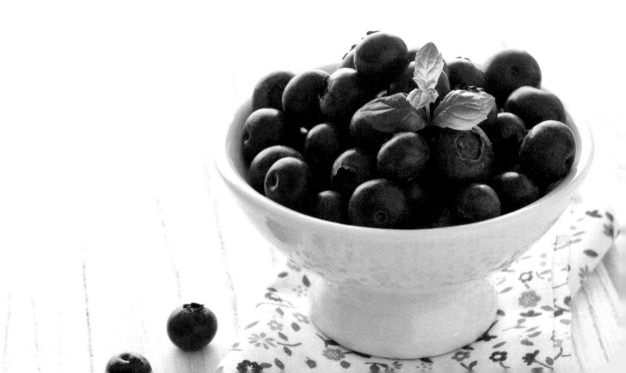

THE AUTHORS

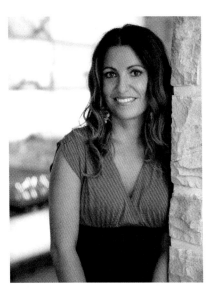

ELISABETH CERQUEIRA

Elisabeth Cerqueira is co-president of NutriSimple, a network of over 50 private nutrition clinics in Quebec. She is the coauthor of the **Superfoods** series and two books in the **Know What To Eat** series: *Weight Loss* and *Arthritis and Inflammation*. She has a bachelor's degree in nutrition from McGill University and is a member of the Ordre professionnel des diététistes du Québec (Professional College of Dietitians of Quebec).

For over 15 years, Elisabeth has been teaching clients to eat by helping them increase the nutritional value of their food. She treats nutritional imbalances that lead to obesity, diabetes, cholesterol, arthritis, anorexia and more. Her mission is to be her clients' partner in health. At the leading edge of scientific research, she and her team of dietitians offer a simple nutritional program. Her empirical approach promotes a diet that helps clients get in peak shape. She is known for her passion for nutrition in medical circles and in the arts. She is a dietitian to a number of celebrities, including Gerard Butler in the movie *300*.

Elisabeth loves to cook with her three children and applies the principles in this book on a daily basis. She believes that eating well should be a simple pleasure. From a European background, she fully enjoys all that life has to offer, including food.

elisabeth@nutrisimple.com
nutrisimple.com

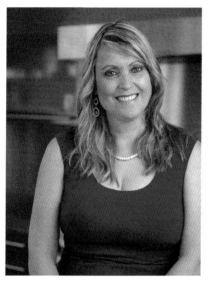

MARISE CHARRON

Marise Charron graduated in nutrition from Laval University and has been a practicing dietitian for over 20 years. She is the author of a number of successful cookbooks and loves to share her knowledge of nutrition and cooking, two related areas that she is passionate about. Marise loves discovering and inventing new recipes and believes that eating well means savoring the moment.

In 1991, Marise founded the Groupe Harmonie Santé to provide professional development to dietitians in private practice and promote discussion among health care professionals. In 2010, she teamed up with Elisabeth Cerqueira to create NutriSimple.

An entrepreneur at heart, she is also at the helm of Nutrition2C (nutrition2c.com), which offers a nutritional analysis and labeling service to companies, schools, restaurants and magazines. In 1998, the Ordre professionnel des diététistes du Québec (Professional College of Dietitians of Quebec) recognized her work with the Annual Merit Award in Nutrition.

As a clinical dietitian, Marise loves the close relationships she develops with her clients, recommending healthy habits using an approach that respects body diversity.

marise@nutrisimple.com
nutrisimple.com

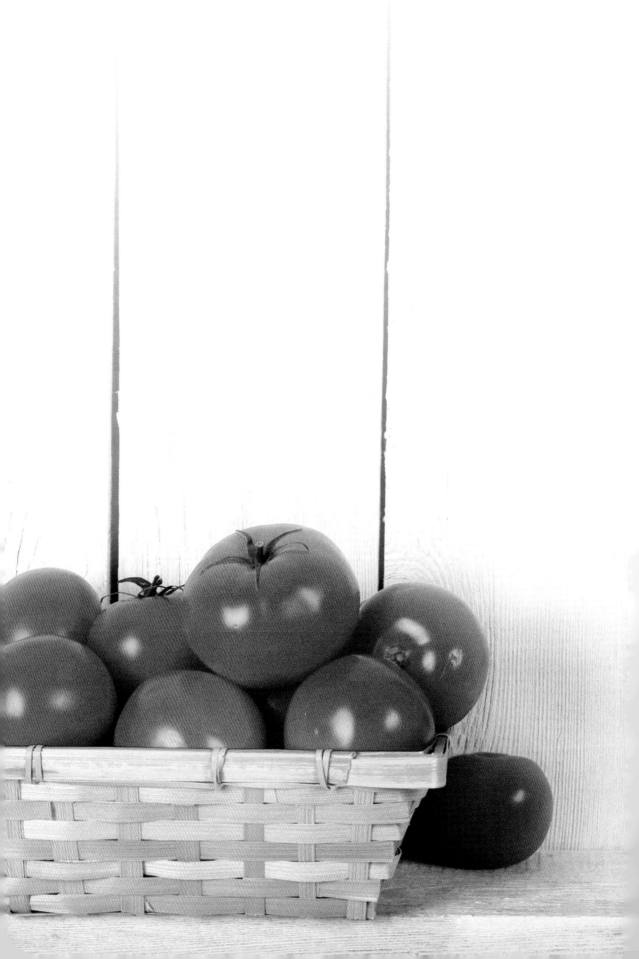

INTRODUCTION

In developed countries, life expectancy at birth increases by approximately three months every year. Given this prolonged life expectancy, it's essential that we learn how to get fit and healthy as early as possible . . . and stay that way for as long as possible.

In this book, we'll teach you how to slow down the effects of aging on your body by adopting a balanced diet. We selected 20 superfoods based on their nutritional value and outlined their virtues for you to discover. By definition, a superfood is a food that possesses more nutrients and health benefits than other foods. Incorporated into a varied and balanced diet, superfoods can provide targeted health benefits. (See note below.)

The superfoods covered in this book are all nutrient-rich and scientifically proven to combat aging. Read through the glossary to learn more about these anti-aging allies. When added to a healthy and balanced diet, these superfoods can improve the skin's elasticity, slow down the appearance of wrinkles, reduce the risk of cardiovascular disease, prevent certain types of cancer, strengthen bones, improve memory and even protect the body against certain degenerative diseases linked to aging such as arthritis, Parkinson's and Alzheimer's.

Preserve your youthfulness by learning how to choose and prepare the right foods — foods that are nutrient-rich and healthy. Discover over 50 healthy recipes that include one or several of the superfoods listed in this book.

And remember — no matter your genetic makeup, a healthy lifestyle and balanced diet can help slow the aging process and have a positive influence on the way in which you age.

NOTE

No one food alone contains all the nutrients a body needs. This is why a healthy, balanced diet is essential for good health. Don't limit your diet to a few superfoods — no matter what their concentration of nutrients — even if they have vitamins and minerals with scientifically proven properties. Include them in your diet, but aim for variety and balance.

LONGEVITY:
THE ESSENTIAL ROLE OF DIET

Free radicals are one of the main mechanisms of the aging process. They are created naturally through processes such as breathing and digestion. In small doses, free radicals are essential to our health and help fight off certain viruses, germs and bacteria and repair damaged cells before they mutate into cancerous ones.

Certain factors can lead to an increase in the production of free radicals. The most common factors include prolonged exposure to sunlight, tobacco use, pollution and emotional and physical stress.

When the body is bombarded by excessive free radicals, it can lead to oxidative stress, an imbalance that can be very damaging to your health. In fact, research shows that when the body overproduces them, free radicals can damage our cells and hinder their ability to regenerate, leading to premature aging.

Free radicals play an important role in many age-related diseases and disorders: atherosclerosis, cataracts, cancer, Alzheimer's, Parkinson's, cardiovascular disease, arthritis, rheumatism and weakening of the immune system.

Free radicals spread through the body by way of a chain reaction: a free radical attacks a molecule and transforms it into another free radical and so on and so forth. As long as the chain reaction is uninterrupted, the free radicals continue to multiply and the damage increases. That's when antioxidants come into play. Antioxidants neutralize free radicals and fight the oxidation process.

Therefore, one of the most effective ways to prevent premature aging is by adopting a balanced diet rich in antioxidants. Antioxidants are mainly found in vitamin C (citrus fruit and berries), vitamin E (nuts, leafy greens), beta-carotene (colorful fruit and vegetables), zinc (seafood, grains), selenium (fish, nuts), omega-3s (oily fish, oils, nuts) and polyphenols (grapes, strawberries).

THE MEDITERRANEAN DIET:
THE SECRET TO A LONG LIFE

Many scientific studies have established a correlation between the diet adopted by the population of the Greek islands of Crete and Corfu and their high life expectancy and low rate of chronic diseases.

THE KEY COMPONENTS OF A MEDITERRANEAN DIET ARE:

• an abundance of fruits and vegetables, garlic, onions, spices and herbs;

• olive oil as a staple fat;

• a daily consumption of legumes, nuts, grains, yogurt and cheese;

• a daily (but moderate) consumption of red wine;

• a higher consumption of fish than chicken or eggs (a few times a week) and a very limited consumption of red meat (a few times a month);

• a limited consumption of processed, sugary foods (a few times a week).

The Mediterranean diet is extremely rich in antioxidants thanks to a very high consumption of fruits, vegetables, legumes and olive oil. Also, because it's plant-based, it's very high in fiber — a major plus when it comes to your intestinal health. With a focus on fish, the Mediterranean diet is low in saturated fat and trans fat, but rich in omega-3s, a powerful fighter against cardiovascular disease. The main sources of protein include fish, legumes, nuts, dairy products, chicken and eggs . . . not red meat. Remember — protein is essential, as it helps develop muscle, which in turn allows us to move. Another important thing to remember: red and processed meat, as well as fatty or sugary products (like commercially baked goods) are linked to a shorter lifespan.

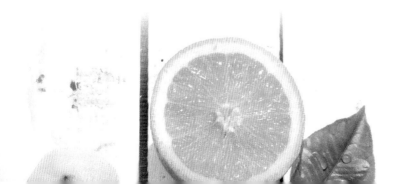

10 TIPS
FOR HEALTHY AGING

1

EAT UNTIL YOU ARE SATIATED — NOT FULL

Don't eat until you're so full you feel like you're about to burst. Try practicing *Hara Hachi Bu* (it literally means "eat until you are 80% full").

HARA HACHI BU: THE OKINAWAN WAY

Hara Hachi Bu means to eat until you are 80% full. The Okinawan people have been practicing this method for centuries, leaving the table almost full, but not entirely. The people of Okinawa are the most long-lived on earth and count among them more centenarians than anywhere else in the world.

Tips for practicing *Hara Hachi Bu*:

- Don't clear your entire plate, stop before and put down your knife and fork.
- Pay attention to your satiation level and ask yourself if the next bite is really necessary.
- If you feel almost full and your hunger begins to wane, get up from the table immediately.

2

EAT FOODS THAT ARE RICH IN OMEGA-3S

Good sources of omega-3s include oily fish, chia seeds, ground flaxseeds and walnuts. Good examples of marine-based sources of fatty acids include salmon, herring, mackerel and sardines.

3

EAT LOTS OF VEGETABLES

Eat an abundance of vegetables on a daily basis (aim to fill approximately half your plate with veggies during main meals and eat about 2 cups/500 ml per day). Vegetables are rich in antioxidants, phytonutrients, vitamins and minerals — all fighters against damage caused by free radicals.

4

ADOPT A MORE VEGETARIAN LIFESTYLE

Cut back on red meat and instead opt for vegetables, legumes, tofu, soy, fruits and nuts. According to several studies, a primarily vegetarian diet helps diminish inflammation.

5 BE PRO PROBIOTIC

Consume lacto-fermented foods like sauerkraut, yogurt, kefir and miso. Probiotics help repopulate good bacteria in your gut and contribute to your intestinal health. If need be, take probiotic supplements (but make sure to follow your dietitian's recommendations).

6 CONSUME FOODS RICH IN SELENIUM

Brazil nuts, salmon and eggs are good examples of foods that are rich in selenium. On top of benefitting the immune system, this antioxidant protects cells against free radicals.

7 DRINK LOTS OF WATER

Proper hydration is the key to stronger joints, improved skin elasticity and overall better health. It's recommended to drink between 4 and 6 cups (1 and 1.5 liters) of water per day.

8 DRINK RED WINE IN MODERATION

In small quantities, red wine is beneficial to your heart. Moderate consumption (1 to 2 glasses per day for women, 2 to 3 glasses per day for men and 1 or 2 alcohol-free days per week — see p. 45) is acceptable, your health permitting.

9 LIMIT YOUR SALT INTAKE

To prevent calcium loss in bones and osteoporosis, do not exceed 2,300 mg of sodium per day — that's the equivalent of 1 teaspoon of salt. Be careful, large quantities of sodium are found in many processed foods sold in supermarkets.

10 ADOPT A HEALTHY LIFESTYLE

Practice strength training and relaxation sports (meditation, yoga, tai chi), go for walks, get 7 to 8 hours of sleep every night, don't smoke, avoid prolonged exposure to the sun and try to maintain a healthy weight.

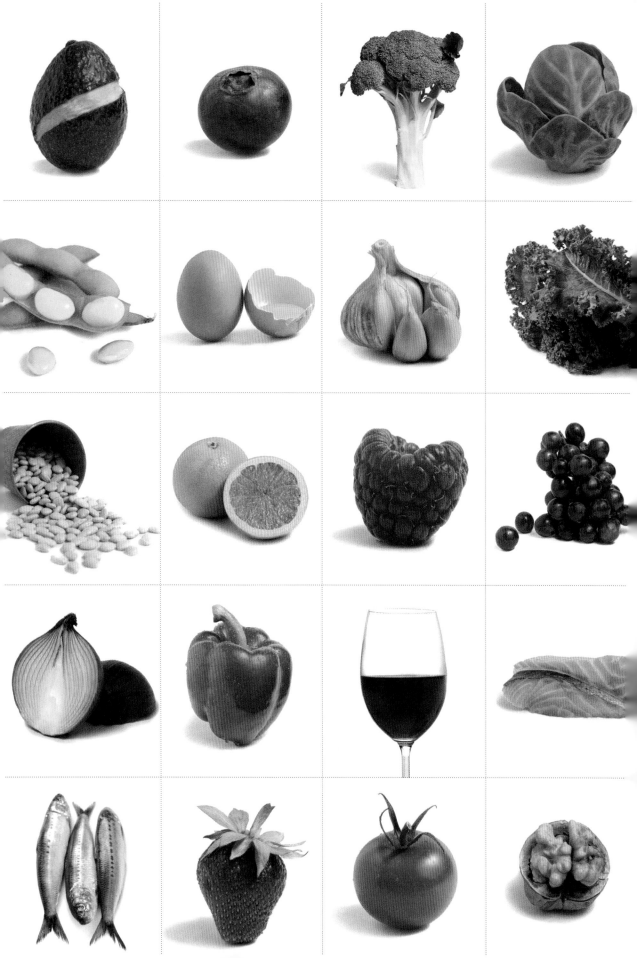

20 SUPERFOODS

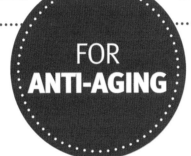

FOR
ANTI-AGING

AVOCADO

Composition

EXCELLENT SOURCE OF: vitamin K, folate, fiber

GOOD SOURCE OF: vitamins B$_5$, B$_6$, C and E

SOURCE OF: copper, magnesium, potassium

Avocados contain tannins, carotenoids
(lutein and zeaxanthin) and phytosterols.

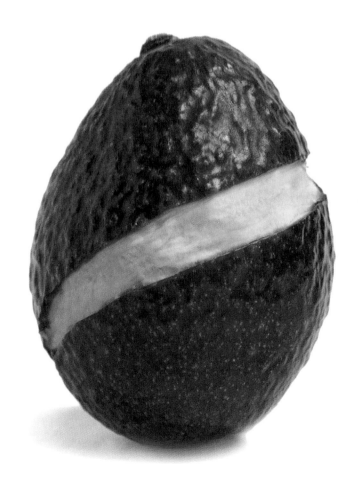

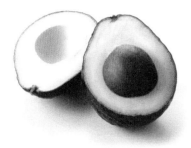

Avocados originate from Central and South America. The word *avocado* comes from the Aztec word *ahuácatl,* meaning "testicle," a reference to its shape and the fact that they typically grow in pairs.

VIRTUES

Improve skin's elasticity
Avocados are extremely nourishing for the skin. A regular consumption of these green powerhouses helps to increase collagen production (collagen is the protein responsible for tissue repair). Collagen helps to prevent wrinkles and other signs of aging, reduces red spots and skin irritations, protects against photoaging caused by the sun and improves skin elasticity and firmness. Plus, the antioxidants found in avocados contribute to the fight against free radicals.

Protect against prostate cancer
Avocados are thought to be able to inhibit the growth of cancerous cells in the prostate. This is probably due to the carotenoids and vitamin E found in the fruit's composition.

Improve cholesterol
Avocados are packed full of heart-healthy fats, fiber and phytosterols — all which help to lower blood cholesterol levels without lowering the body's HDL cholesterol level (the "good" cholesterol). And that means a healthy heart and a longer life.

Reduce the risk of macular degeneration
The carotenoids found in avocados play a key role in eye health and help reduce the risk of macular degeneration, an age-related eye disease.

THINGS TO REMEMBER

• One avocado contains almost as many antioxidants as ½ cup (125 ml) of broccoli.

• Unlike other sources of fat, avocados contain both soluble and insoluble fiber. Soluble fiber helps stabilize blood sugar and insoluble fiber regulates bowel health and helps make you feel fuller longer.

HOW TO EAT IT

• As a guacamole or mousse, in smoothies, salads and sandwiches.

• Stuffed with seafood or chicken.

─────── **DID YOU KNOW?** ───────

An avocado's color is indicative of its variety and not its level of ripeness. However, if the skin near the stem is very dark, the fruit is most likely overripe.

BLUEBERRIES

Composition

GOOD SOURCE OF: vitamin K, fiber
SOURCE OF: vitamins C and E, manganese

Blueberries are high in antioxidants
(including flavonoids and phenolic acids).

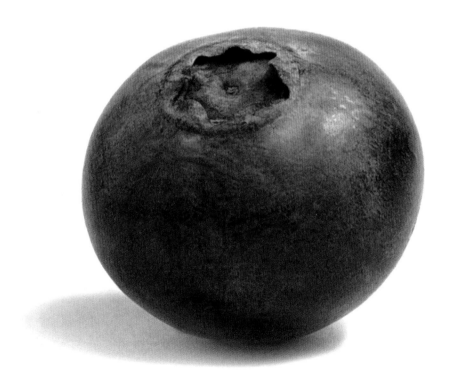

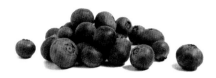

Blueberries (and their European cousins, bilberries) started growing in North America and Eurasia hundreds of years ago. However, it wasn't until the early twentieth century that they began being cultivated all over the world.

VIRTUES

Help combat free radicals
Of all the berries, blueberries have the highest antioxidant count.

Help prevent cancer
A regular consumption of blueberries has been shown to help prevent certain aggressive, even fatal, breast cancers. A 132-lb (60 kg) woman should eat ¾ cup (180 ml) of fresh blueberries every day.

Lower the risk of cardiovascular disease
The phenolic acids and flavonoids found in blueberries help prevent oxidation of LDL cholesterol (the "bad" cholesterol) and diminish inflammation of the vascular system, which in turn helps to lower the risk of cardiovascular disease.

Help improve memory
Blueberries improve memory and slow down the cognitive decline associated with Alzheimer's and Parkinson's.

THINGS TO REMEMBER

Anthocyanin, the pigment that makes blueberries blue, is one of the most beneficial antioxidants when it comes to preventing age-related diseases.

HOW TO EAT IT

• On their own, as a jam or jelly, with cereal or rolled oats, in a smoothie, on pancakes (buckwheat or oat bran), in a ricotta verrine, with frozen yogurt or sorbet.

• As a coulis, served with halibut, poultry or pork tenderloin.

─────── **BLUEBERRIES: FRESH OR FROZEN?** ───────

Frozen blueberries don't contain as much vitamin C as fresh blueberries, but they're just as rich in antioxidants. Because blueberry season is so short, buy your berries in large quantities, freeze them on a cookie sheet and then place into freezer bags — ready to use whenever you want!

BROCCOLI

Composition

EXCELLENT SOURCE OF: vitamins C and K

SOURCE OF: vitamins A, B_2, B_5, B_6 and E, magnesium, manganese, copper, phosphorus, potassium, folate, fiber

Broccoli contains sulfur compounds (isothiocyanates) and carotenoids (lutein and zeaxanthin).

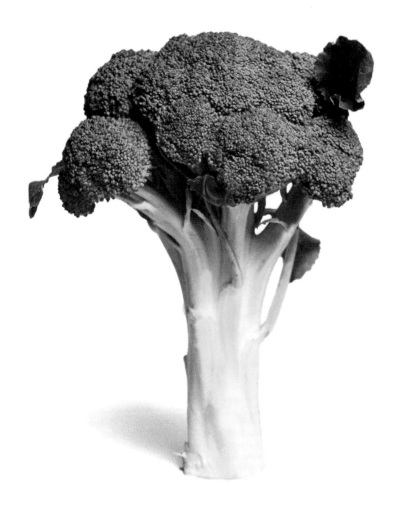

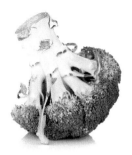

Because of its popularity in Mediterranean cuisine, broccoli, the most nutrient-dense vegetable on the planet, is often referred to as "Italian asparagus."

VIRTUES

Diminishes the risk of cardiovascular disease
A regular consumption of broccoli (at least five times a week) has been shown to considerably reduce the risk of heart-related death.

Prevents eye disease
The carotenoids found in broccoli help prevent macular degeneration and cataracts.

Lowers the risk of cancer
Eating 3 to 5 portions of broccoli a week helps lower your risk of cancer, especially ovarian and prostate cancers.

Fights the signs of aging
Broccoli is packed with provitamin A, an anti-aging carotenoid that keeps the skin looking young.

THINGS TO REMEMBER

• Munching on raw broccoli is the best way to benefit from all its nutritional goodness. When heated, broccoli loses some of its nutrients.

• When preparing broccoli, make sure to limit its cooking time (between 5 and 7 minutes). To quickly halt the cooking process, immediately remove the florets from the heat and pass them under cold water or plunge them into an ice bath.

HOW TO EAT IT

Raw: in a salad or served with dip.

Cooked: in a soup, puréed with potatoes, au gratin, in soufflés, flans, quiches and stir-fries.

─────── **SOMETHING TO DISCOVER** ───────

We tend to eat only the florets, but did you know that broccoli stalks are just as delicious? Peel and cut them into sticks, then steam or cook them in the oven for 8 to 10 minutes until tender. Eat them just as you would asparagus, with a side of vinaigrette or mayonnaise.

BRUSSELS SPROUTS

EXCELLENT SOURCE OF: vitamins C and K

GOOD SOURCE OF: folate, fiber

SOURCE OF: vitamins A, B_1, B_2, B_6 and E, iron, potassium, manganese, magnesium, copper, phosphorus

Brussels sprouts contain sulfur compounds (isothiocyanates) and carotenoids (lutein and zeaxanthin).

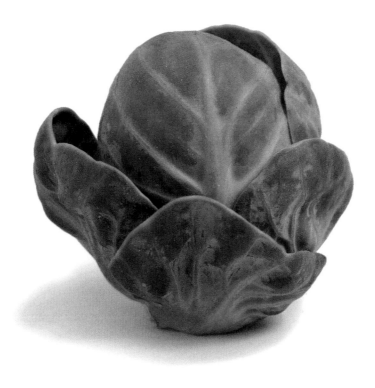

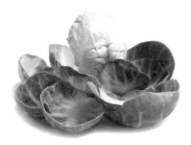

Brussels sprouts are so called because they were first introduced in Brussels, Belgium, near the end of the twelfth century. In the seventeenth century, following a massive increase in the cultivation of vegetables, the buds of this tiny cabbage began growing along the length of fibrous stalks.

VIRTUES

Reduce the risk of certain types of cancer
Like other cruciferous vegetables, Brussels sprouts contain sulfur compounds. A regular consumption (at least three times a week) has been shown to significantly reduce (up to 50%) the risk of developing certain types of cancer, including lung, bladder, gastro-intestinal and breast cancers.

Protect against rheumatoid arthritis
Brussels sprouts are high in vitamin C, which may help protect against rheumatoid arthritis.

Help prevent cataracts
When eaten regularly, the carotenoids found in Brussels sprouts have been shown to prevent macular degeneration.

THINGS TO REMEMBER
1 cup (250 ml) of Brussels sprouts contains 200% of the recommended daily intake of vitamin K, 150% of the recommended daily intake of vitamin C and 25% of the recommended daily intake of vitamin A and folate.

COOKING
• It's best to steam Brussels sprouts, as their compounds are extremely soluble in water. However, if you prefer cooking them directly in water, here's how to make sure you're still getting the most out of their nutritional value: Cut the sprouts in two (this will reduce cooking time). Next, bring a pot of water to a boil and drop the sprouts in. Let simmer uncovered on medium-low heat for 6 to 7 minutes.

• To minimize the smell, drop a walnut (still in its shell), a celery stalk or a crouton of bread into the boiling water.

HOW TO EAT IT
• In the form of chips.

• As a side dish, roasted in the oven, incorporated into mashed potatoes or au gratin.

EDAMAME

Composition

EXCELLENT SOURCE OF: vitamins B_2 and K, copper, manganese, magnesium, omega-3 fatty acids

GOOD SOURCE OF: protein, fiber, vitamins B_1 and B_6, folate, zinc, selenium, iron

SOURCE OF: calcium, vitamins B_5, C and E

Edamame contain beta-carotene and flavonoids (including quercetin).

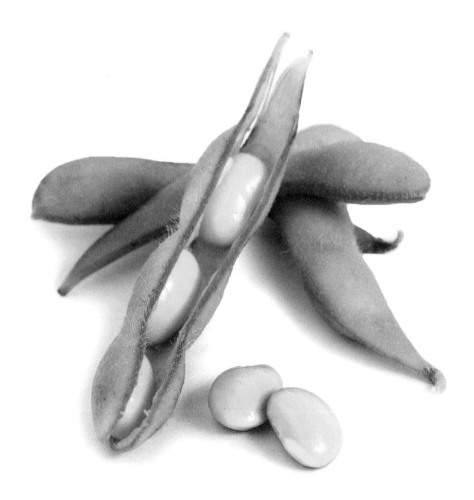

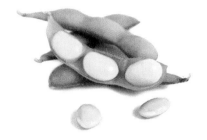

This green soybean hails from Asia. Edamame means "twig bean" in Japanese. Although these protein-packed beans can be cooked like a vegetable, they're in fact part of the legume family.

VIRTUES

Prevent wrinkles

The flavonoids that are so abundant in edamame help prevent wrinkles. They protect the skin's collagen from damage caused by UV rays and act as antioxidants that help neutralize the free radicals produced as a result of sun exposure.

Reduce the risks of cardiovascular disease

The consumption of edamame helps lower total cholesterol and blood pressure, two at-risk factors when it comes to cardiovascular disease. Plus, it helps prevent heart attacks and strokes.

Increase bone density

Edamame beans are loaded with nutrients such as vitamin K, manganese, magnesium and phosphorus, which help strengthen bones and build bone density.

Prevent cancer

Eating ¼ cup (60 ml) of edamame per day is sufficient to benefit from the anticancer flavonoids found in them.

THINGS TO REMEMBER

• Edamame pack a protein punch that is more powerful than any other legume.

• 1 cup (250 ml) of boiled edamame contains 24 g of protein — that's more protein than 3 oz (90 g) of meat, chicken or fish.

• Edamame contain more flavonoids than other soy products (such as tofu).

HOW TO EAT IT

• As a snack or in a purée (like hummus).

• In soups, salads, Asian stir-fries.

──────── **SOMETHING TO DISCOVER** ────────

For a unique appetizer, blanch or sauté a handful of edamame beans (still in their pods) for 3 to 4 minutes and serve them with a sprinkling of sea salt. (The pods are not edible.)

EGGS

Composition

EXCELLENT SOURCE OF: selenium, choline

GOOD SOURCE OF: vitamins B_2, B_8 and B_{12}

SOURCE OF: vitamins A, B_5, D and E, folate, phosphorus, zinc, protein

Eggs contain carotenoids (lutein and zeaxanthin).

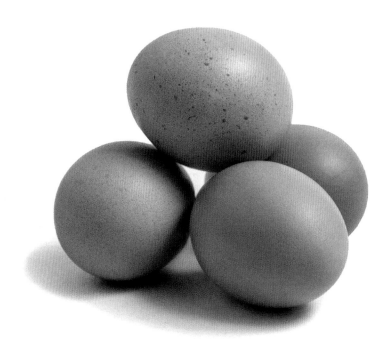

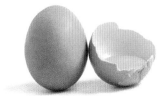

The first written record of humans eating chicken eggs dates back to 1200 BC with the Egyptians and the Chinese.

VIRTUES

Improve memory
Choline, a micronutrient abundant in eggs, promotes brain health and improves memory.

Protect the skin
Egg yolk contains carotenoids, which help protect the skin against harmful UV rays.

Prevent cataracts
According to several studies, the carotenoids found in egg yolk help reduce the risk of macular degeneration. The body absorbs the carotenoids found in eggs more easily than the carotenoids found in carrots or spinach because of the yolk's fatty content.

Protect against breast cancer
The high levels of lutein and zeaxanthin (the two main carotenoids found in eggs) have been shown to reduce the risk of breast cancer in postmenopausal women.

THINGS TO REMEMBER

• Eggs are considered complete proteins because they contain all the essential amino acids.

• Watch out for salmonella, bacteria that causes food poisoning. While the risk is minimal, only eat raw or undercooked eggs (for example, in mayonnaise, egg vinaigrette or in a mousse for dessert) if you are sure they are fresh and pasteurized.

• The inside of the egg must not come in contact with the outside of the shell to avoid any risk of contamination.

STORING

To properly store eggs, keep them on a shelf in the refrigerator and not on the door, preferably in their box so that you know the expiry date. Eggs should be placed tips down. They will keep this way for about three weeks. To find out whether an egg is fresh, dunk it in a saucepan of water. If it sinks, it's fresh; if it floats, it's too old to eat.

HOW TO EAT IT

• Poached, hard-boiled, soft-boiled, scrambled, sunny side up, in salads and sandwiches.

• In omelets, frittatas, soufflés, quiches, crêpes and cakes.

• For making pasta and thickening sauces.

DID YOU KNOW?

The color of the shell (white or brown) has no bearing on the nutritional value of eggs and depends exclusively on the type of chicken.

GARLIC

Composition

GOOD SOURCE OF: magnesium, vitamin B_6

SOURCE OF: copper, selenium

Garlic contains sulfur compounds
and flavonoids (including quercetin).

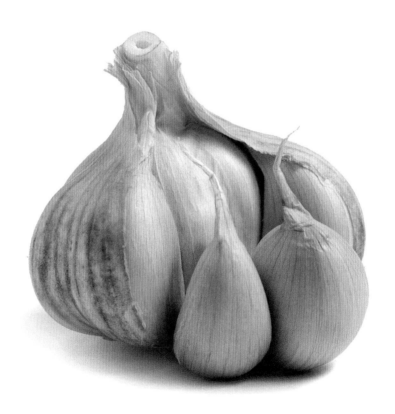

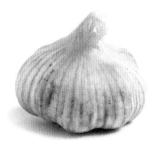

Garlic has been used for its therapeutic properties since Antiquity. In addition to its anti-inflammatory, antiseptic, antifungal and cholesterol-lowering properties, it helps lower blood pressure, acts as a blood thinner and fights cancer — a veritable panacea. Garlic's reputation has definitely stood the test of time.

VIRTUES

Helps prevent digestive cancers

A regular consumption of garlic (6 cooked or raw cloves per week) is believed to help prevent certain types of cancer, notably digestive cancer. In fact, the molecules that are released when garlic is crushed have the ability to stop the growth of cancerous cells, in some cases eradicating them altogether.

Improves cholesterol

Eating garlic on a daily basis is thought to lower total cholesterol, LDL cholesterol (the "bad" cholesterol) and triglycerides (fat that circulates in the bloodstream), which are all culprits when it comes to cardiovascular disease.

THINGS TO REMEMBER

• To actually benefit from garlic's therapeutic effects, you need to eat at least one fresh garlic clove per day (chopped or crushed). To help your body absorb the active compounds, eat your raw garlic with a bit of olive oil.

• When cooking with garlic, crush the cloves and let them sit 10 minutes before using them. This helps produce the compound allicin, which in itself boasts many virtues.

• The best way to consume garlic is raw; raw garlic is far more beneficial than cooked garlic. Heat destroys the healthy sulfur compounds that are so good for you. When cooking, add garlic only near the end of the cooking process (the last 20 minutes or so). And finally, remember that the finer it's chopped, the stronger it tastes!

STORING

Store garlic in a dark, dry, well-ventilated place. Garlic is best stored at room temperature; the cold from the refrigerator will trigger germination.

HOW TO EAT IT

Raw: in aïoli, bruschetta, pesto, vinaigrette or marinade.

Cooked: confit, sautéed with vegetables, in soups and sauces.

─────── DID YOU KNOW? ───────

Eating garlic while breastfeeding can change the taste and smell of breast milk.

KALE

Composition

EXCELLENT SOURCE OF: vitamins A, C and K, manganese

GOOD SOURCE OF: copper, calcium, fiber

SOURCE OF: vitamins B_1, B_2, B_3, B_6 and E, folate, potassium, magnesium

Kale contains beta-carotene, carotenoids (lutein and zeaxanthin), flavonoids (including quercetin) and sulfur compounds (isothiocyanates).

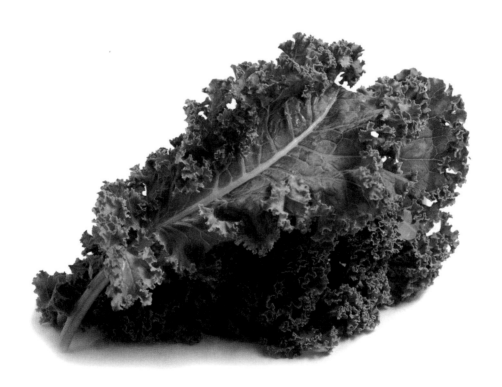

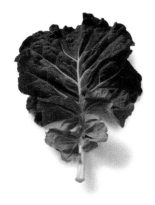

There are several different types of kale (Curly, Lacinato, Red Russian, etc.), and they vary in color and size. Kale leaves do not form a tight head, but instead branch off from a central stem.

VIRTUES

Protects against the signs of aging
Kale boasts an impressive number of flavonoids and other antioxidants that help protect the body against free radicals, one of the biggest culprits when it comes to aging.

Protects against certain types of cancer
Eating kale at least three times a week is believed to lower the risk of certain types of cancer (bladder, breast, ovarian, prostate and colon). Plus, its high level of beta-carotene helps prevent skin cancer.

Helps prevent cataracts
The carotenoids found in kale help lower the risk of cataracts, macular degeneration and glaucoma. Cataracts and macular degeneration are often linked to aging.

Helps maintain a healthy cardiovascular system
Kale is a great ally in the fight against cardiovascular disease. A regular consumption of this leafy green helps lower cholesterol and reduces inflammation of the blood vessels.

THINGS TO REMEMBER

• Kale is loaded with twice the level of antioxidants contained in other leafy greens.

• Kale contains eight times the recommended daily intake of vitamin K and double the recommended daily intake of vitamin A.

STORING

Pat the leaves dry with a paper towel, being careful not to damage the center rib. Store the leaves in a loosely closed freezer bag and keep in the coolest part of the refrigerator. When stored like this, kale can last up to two weeks. However, the sooner you eat it, the less bitter it will taste.

HOW TO EAT IT

The most popular part of kale is the leaf itself — the stalk and rib are rather fibrous.

Raw: in smoothies, salads, tabbouleh and wraps.

Cooked: in the form of chips, in soups, omelets, stews or simply sautéed in a skillet with a drizzle of olive oil and some garlic and served as a side dish.

LIMA BEANS

Composition

EXCELLENT SOURCE OF: molybdenum, copper, manganese, folate, vitamin B_1, fiber

GOOD SOURCE OF: iron, magnesium, vitamins B_6 and B_5, zinc, selenium, potassium, phosphorus

SOURCE OF: vitamins B_2, C, E and K, protein

Lima beans contain phytosterols.

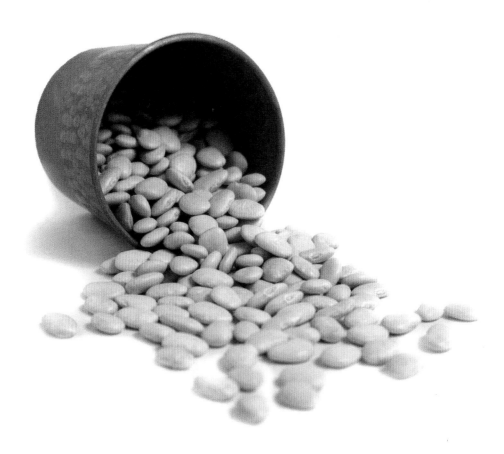

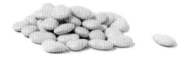

Lima beans belong to the legume family. Although Guatemala appears to be their country of origin, lima beans mainly come from South America, where they are named after the capital of Peru.

VIRTUES

Good for the skin
Packed with a wide range of minerals and trace elements, lima beans help keep skin healthy and protect skin cells from the effects of premature aging.

Lower the risk of a heart attack
A major study conducted over the course of 25 years in seven different countries suggests that a high level of legume consumption (i.e., lima beans) can help reduce the risk of a fatal heart attack by as much as 82%. This is in large part due to the high levels of fiber found in lima beans.

Lower the risk of colon cancer
According to a study involving 2,000 individuals having been diagnosed with colon cancer, those who adopted a diet high in legumes were 65% less likely to experience a relapse, even if theirs was an advanced-stage cancer.

THINGS TO REMEMBER
• The nutritional value of canned beans is about the same as dried beans. However, it's important to thoroughly rinse canned beans prior to consuming them to reduce your sodium intake and risk of flatulence.

• It's recommended that those who eat little or no animal protein combine legumes with grains or nuts. Combined, these two incomplete proteins means you're getting a complete protein (which provides us with essential amino acids). For children, adolescents, pregnant women and seniors each meal must include a complete protein — everyone else can load up on their proteins however they see fit.

SOAKING
If you prefer buying dried beans, it's important to leave them soaking in the refrigerator overnight (make sure you change the water once or twice), cook them thoroughly and rinse abundantly once they're done. If you are bothered by flatulence, we recommend quickly soaking lima beans before consuming them (p. 173).

HOW TO EAT IT
• In a soup or salad.

• As a side dish, boiled and served with a knob of butter.

——— SOMETHING TO DISCOVER ———
Lima bean purée is similar to chickpea hummus. To prepare it, simply purée the lima beans with a drizzle of olive oil and lemon juice. Add chopped parsley and mix.

PINK GRAPEFRUIT

Composition

EXCELLENT SOURCE OF: vitamin C

GOOD SOURCE OF: vitamin A (in the form of beta-carotene)

SOURCE OF: folate, vitamin B_1, potassium, magnesium,
soluble fiber (especially pectin)

Pink grapefruit contains carotenoids,
flavonoids and limonoids.

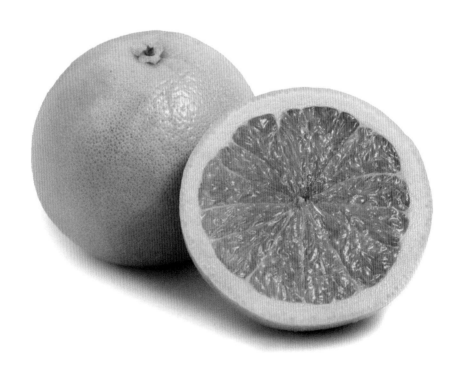

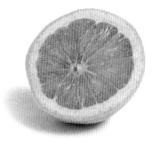

The citrus fruit known as grapefruit is in fact a pomelo. A pink grapefruit is a cross between an orange and a pomelo.

VIRTUES

Promotes healthy skin
Grapefruit is bursting with vitamin C, which is responsible for the synthesis of collagen, which in turn is responsible for the skin's elasticity.

Prevents certain cancers
Eating grapefruit between one and four times a week has been shown to prevent prostate, stomach and colorectal cancer, as well as cancer of the oral cavity, larynx, pharynx and esophagus. This is mainly due to the high levels of antioxidants and limonoids found in this citrus powerhouse.

Lowers cholesterol
Grapefruit contains a high concentration of polyphenols, vitamin C and pectin, which all help to significantly lower blood lipid levels.

THINGS TO REMEMBER

• There are a variety of different grapefruit, including white, pink and red. The pink and red varieties are the most beneficial to your health, as they owe their color to lycopene, an antioxidant that boasts cancer-fighting properties.

• Fresh grapefruit offers a much higher concentration of nutrients (namely flavonoids and soluble fiber) than store-bought grapefruit juice.

• Be careful! Grapefruit can interact with certain medications and lead to adverse side effects. A single glass of grapefruit juice taken while on some medications can cause serious complications for up to three days following consumption. Potential interactions are indicated on a medication's label.

HOW TO EAT IT

• Cut in segments and tossed into a fruit salad, grilled with a drizzle of maple syrup, in a sorbet or as a granita.

• Juiced, served as a drink or used in a vinaigrette or marinade.

─── **DID YOU KNOW?** ───

Grapefruit is at its sweetest and most flavorful between November and January (peak harvesting season). It's recommended to take grapefruit out of the refrigerator a few hours prior to eating it (or the night before if you intend to serve it for breakfast), as it becomes even juicier at room temperature.

RASPBERRIES

Composition

EXCELLENT SOURCE OF: vitamin C, fiber
GOOD SOURCE OF: manganese
SOURCE OF: vitamins E and K, folate, iron, magnesium, potassium

Raspberries contain phenolic acids,
flavonoids and tannins.

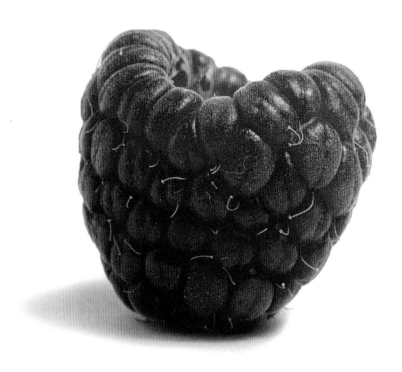

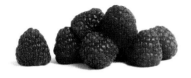

Raspberries have been harvested for millennia (long before scientific research started looking into their benefits) and sought after for their numerous medicinal qualities, notably their ability to fight fatigue and ease constipation.

VIRTUES

Reduce the risk of cardiovascular disease
The phenolic acids found in raspberries help lower the risk of cardiovascular disease, notably by stopping the oxidation of LDL cholesterol (the "bad" cholesterol).

Protect against the proliferation of cancerous cells
Raspberries are the second most powerful cancer-fighting berry in the world (first place goes to blueberries); they help prevent cancerous cells and tumors from multiplying.

Slow down the aging process
A regular consumption of raspberries helps protect the skin against photoaging. In fact, the flavonoids present in raspberries help trigger a protective reaction against inflammation of the skin caused by UV rays, which could lead to skin cancer.

Contribute to cognitive health
Raspberries are bursting with antioxidants which are known for protecting the brain's cells from becoming damaged by free radicals. This leads to a better connection between neurons, which in turn help to improve cognitive skills.

THINGS TO REMEMBER

• The redder the raspberry, the richer it is in antioxidants.

• Twenty raspberries contain 7.4 g of dietary fiber — that's close to a third of the recommended daily intake!

HOW TO EAT IT

• In cereal, oatmeal or smoothies.

• In mixed salads and fruit salads.

• As a pancake or waffle topper, in muffins, yogurt, with chocolate fondue, in coulis, sorbet, Popsicle or mousse form, in a clafouti.

RED GRAPES

Composition

GOOD SOURCE OF: vitamin K, manganese

SOURCE OF: copper, vitamins B_1, B_6 and C, potassium

Grapes contain flavonoids, phenolic acids, carotenoids and resveratrol.

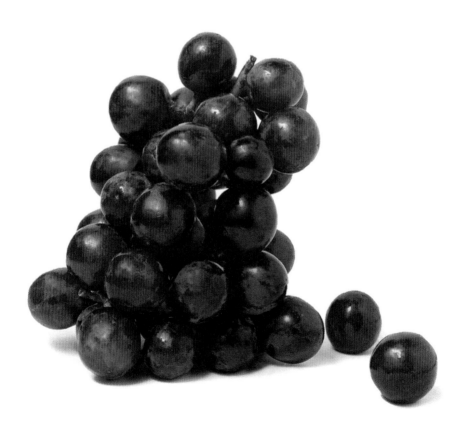

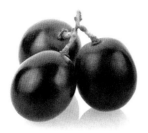

Grapes have been revered for their numerous virtues since Antiquity, believed to be the miracle remedy for constipation, gout, arthritis and skin conditions.

VIRTUES

Improve skin's elasticity
Red grapes are rich in flavonoids, which promote collagen and elastin production, which in turn helps improve the skin's elasticity. Flavonoids also protect the body against free radicals, which are responsible for cell damage and aging of the skin.

Prevent cardiovascular disease
The resveratrol and flavonoids found in grapes have been shown to have beneficial effects on the body's cardiovascular health, namely improving blood cell elasticity, reducing oxidation of LDL cholesterol (the "bad" cholesterol), increasing HDL cholesterol levels (the "good" cholesterol), preventing the formation of blood clots and lowering blood pressure.

Help fight memory loss
A daily consumption of 2 cups (500 ml) of red grape juice has been shown to improve the cognitive functions of individuals suffering from memory loss non-related to Alzheimer's.

THINGS TO REMEMBER
• Red grapes have twice as many antioxidants as green grapes. This is due to the high levels of flavonoids that give red grapes their bright color.

• Red grapes are one of the best sources of resveratrol, a good ally in the fight against cancer and aging.

• You can also consume grapes in the form of juice or wine (as long as you moderate your consumption — see p. 45).

HOW TO EAT IT
• On cheese platters or in a salad.

• In juice form, in fruit salads, as garnish on cakes, waffles or pancakes, in jelly or jam form.

─── **SOMETHING TO DISCOVER** ───

Freeze grapes on a cookie sheet. Once they're completely frozen, transfer them to a freezer bag and continue to store them in the freezer until ready to enjoy. Use them in your desserts or pop them in your mouth for a sweet (low-cal) snack.

RED ONIONS

Composition

SOURCE OF: folate, fiber, vitamins B_6 and C, manganese, potassium

Red onions contain selenium, flavonoids (including quercetin) and sulfur compounds (isothiocyanates).

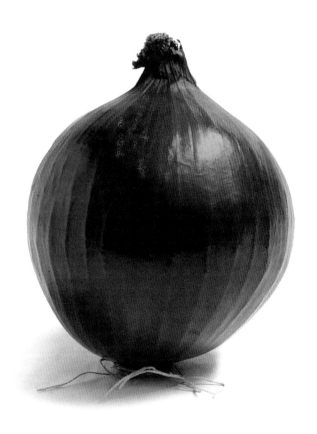

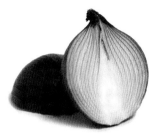

Onions are among the oldest known cultivated plants. For eons now they've been used for their medicinal properties and are believed to help prevent hair loss, fight off infections and eliminate cellulite.

VIRTUES

Reduce the risk of certain cancers
Eating between 1 and 7 servings of red onions per week (approximately ⅓ cup/80 ml of cooked onion per serving) has been shown to reduce the risk of certain cancers, notably colorectal and ovarian and cancer of the oral cavity, larynx, esophagus and pharynx.

Improve cardiovascular health
The flavonoids present in red onions help protect blood vessels and can even prevent heart attacks. The synergetic interaction they form with the sulfur compounds has been shown to reduce platelet aggregation, a condition that can lead to blood clots such as deep vein thrombosis.

Fight the aging process
The many antioxidants found in onions help protect the body's cells from the damages caused by free radicals.

THINGS TO REMEMBER
• Red onions are much richer in antioxidants than paler onions.

• Cooked onion is richer in antioxidants than raw onion. The quercetin found in onions is very beneficial, withstands heat and is easier for the body to absorb once cooked. So, raw or cooked? Although heat destroys some of the vitamins, cooked onion is better.

STORING
• Store onions in a cool, dry place, away from light.

• Do not leave a cut onion out in the open. Not only will it lose some of its vitamins and minerals, but it runs the risk of becoming toxic due to the oxidation process. Instead, slice leftover onions and store in the freezer for future use.

HOW TO EAT IT
Raw: in salads and hamburgers.

Cooked: confit, sautéed with vegetables, in soups, quiches and on pizzas.

RED PEPPER

Composition

EXCELLENT SOURCE OF: vitamins A and C
GOOD SOURCE OF: vitamin B_6, folate
SOURCE OF: fiber, potassium, vitamins B_2 and B_5
Red peppers contain carotenoids
(including beta-carotene, lycopene and capsanthin).

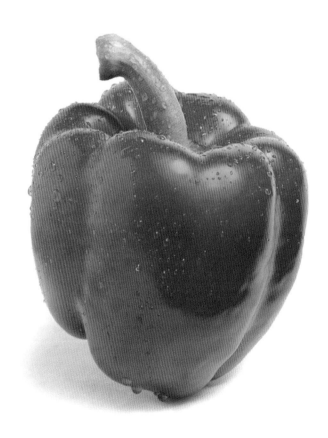

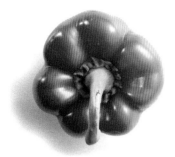

From a cooking standpoint, there exist two main categories of peppers: hot peppers, which are used as spice, and sweet peppers, which are consumed like vegetables.

VIRTUES

Prevent cancer
Munching on peppers could diminish the risk of cancer, as they're loaded with cancer-fighting properties like vitamin C and carotenoids.

Protect and repair skin cells
The carotenoids (such as capsanthin) found in red peppers offer increased protection against damages caused by pollution and UV rays. As for the vitamin C, it's essential to the production of collagen and repairs DNA damaged by the sun.

Prevent degenerative diseases
Red peppers are packed with vitamin C, which helps diminish oxidation and inflammation throughout the body, protecting against degenerative diseases linked to aging (like arthritis and Alzheimer's and Parkinson's).

THINGS TO REMEMBER

• In equal volume, red peppers pack more vitamin C than citrus fruit.

• Red peppers contain one and a half times more vitamin C and nine times more vitamin A than green peppers.

• To benefit from a higher dose of vitamin C, it's best to consume red peppers raw, rather than cooked.

• The fresher the pepper, the richer it is in nutrients. Look for peppers that are firm and heavy with taut skin; avoid peppers with wrinkles and spots.

HOW TO EAT IT

Raw: with dip or in a salad.

Cooked: roasted, grilled, stuffed, in soups, stir-fries, chili, fajitas and frittatas.

─── **DID YOU KNOW?** ───

Depending on its stage of maturity, a pepper will change colors, from green to yellow to red. Once it's been harvested, however, it will cease changing colors.

RED WINE

Composition

SOURCE OF: magnesium

Wine is very rich in polyphenols (including resveratrol).

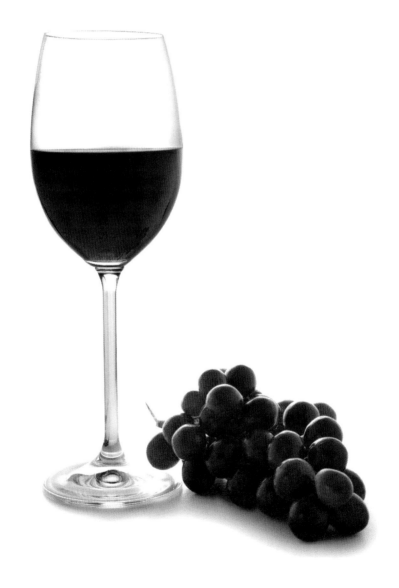

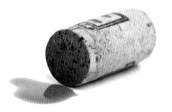

It is estimated that winemaking dates back over 5,000 years. At the beginning of the third millennium BC, the Egyptians were busy domesticating grapevines, while the Chinese were mastering the art of winemaking.

VIRTUES

Increases life expectancy and improves quality of life
Red wine, when consumed in moderation, has been shown to lower the risk of chronic illness. A moderate consumption of wine could increase life expectancy — reducing the risk of all-cause mortality by 20 to 30% — in addition to fighting off Alzheimer's and slowing down cognitive decline by as much as 85%.

Slows down the aging process
The resveratrol present in wine has been shown to reverse damage to the skin caused by UV rays. In fact, this powerful antioxidant is actually capable of blocking the damaging effects free radicals can potentially have on the epidermis.

Lowers the risk of cardiovascular disease
Alcohol and resveratrol have anti-inflammatory properties that help lower the risk of cardiovascular disease in older men and women. A moderate consumption of alcohol, taken on a regular basis as opposed to binge drinking, has been shown to increase HDL cholesterol (the "good" cholesterol). Plus, red wine helps thin the blood and prevent platelet aggregation from occurring, thus lowering the risk of heart disease and stroke.

THINGS TO REMEMBER

• You would need to consume much more grape juice than wine to benefit from the same protective effects. Fermentation helps with the production of resveratrol and the alcohol helps with its absorption.

• The alcohol content in wine is thought to increase good cholesterol.

• When consumed in too-large quantities, red wine loses all its health benefits, namely by affecting cognitive functions and increasing the risk of cancer. Alcohol abuse can reduce life expectancy by up to two years.

HOW TO CONSUME IT

• As a beverage, served with a meal.

• To deglaze a skillet or as a marinade for meat.

—— MODERATION GUIDELINE ——

Women: 1 to 2 drinks a day and 1 to 2 alcohol-free days every week
Men: 2 to 3 drinks a day and 1 to 2 alcohol-free days every week

One drink is equal to:
• 1 glass of beer (12 oz/340 ml, 5% alcohol)
• 1 glass of fortified wine (3 oz/85 ml, 20% alcohol)
• 1 glass of wine (5 oz/140 ml, 12% alcohol)
• 1 shot of spirits (1½ oz/45 ml, 40% alcohol)

SALMON

Composition

EXCELLENT SOURCE OF: omega-3 fatty acids, protein, phosphorus, selenium, vitamins B_1, B_3, B_5, B_6, B_{12} and D

GOOD SOURCE OF: potassium

SOURCE OF: magnesium, zinc, copper, folate, vitamin B_2, iron

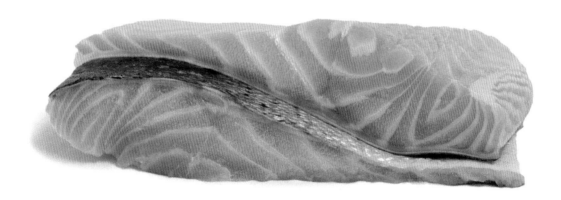

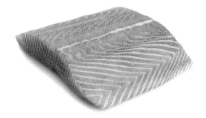

The term *salmon* is used to describe several of the species belonging to the Salmonidae family. These ocean or freshwater fish live mainly in the northern Atlantic and Pacific oceans. The salmon found in the markets is largely farmed.

VIRTUES

Reduces the risk of cardiovascular disease
Eating 3 oz (90 g) of salmon every week has been shown to diminish the risk of a heart attack by approximately 70%.

Prevents cognitive decline
Several studies have shown that certain omega-3 fatty acids can help slow down the cognitive decline in people suffering from mild cognitive impairment.

Reduces inflammation
The Arthritis Society recommends that those suffering from inflammatory arthritis (with the exception of gout) eat fish rich in omega-3s twice a week.

Improves skin
According to several studies, certain omega-3 fatty acids could play a role in preventing and treating skin aging caused by the sun's rays.

Prevents osteoporosis
Salmon is an excellent source of vitamin D, which plays a key role in helping bones absorb calcium the body needs. Eating salmon twice a week has been shown to help prevent osteoporosis. Eating canned fish, including the bones (with caution), helps increase calcium levels.

THINGS TO REMEMBER

Salmon is one of the best sources of omega-3 fatty acids, which reduce the risk of cardiovascular disease. However, the quantity of omega-3s varies depending on the species; salmon from the Atlantic boasts the highest level of omega-3s.

HOW TO EAT IT

Raw: gravlax, tartare, ceviche or sashimi.

Cooked: grilled, poached or smoked.

———— SALMON: CANNED OR FRESH? ————

Whether it's canned or fresh, salmon's nutritional value is pretty much the same. However, canned salmon contains more sodium. Pound for pound, canned salmon (wild salmon) can contain up to eight times more sodium and slightly lower omega-3 levels than fresh salmon (farmed salmon). But don't forget: canned salmon allows you to up your calcium intake if you eat the fish whole, bones and all.

SARDINES

Composition

EXCELLENT SOURCE OF: protein, omega-3 fatty acids, calcium, selenium, vitamins B$_3$, B$_{12}$ and D, phosphorus
GOOD SOURCE OF: iron, copper, vitamin B$_2$
SOURCE OF: zinc, potassium

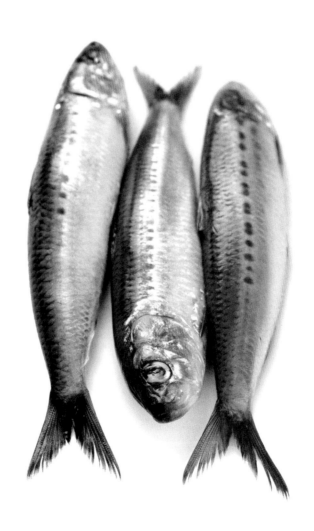

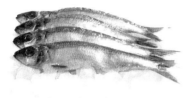

The word *sardine* comes from the Latin *Sardae sine sardinae*, which means "fish of Sardinia." Fished off the Mediterranean coast for centuries, sardines are a staple in Italian and Portuguese cuisine. The word *sardine* refers to not just one fish, but some 20 varieties of small fish.

VIRTUES

Reduce the risk of cardiovascular disease
Sardines are rich in omega-3 fatty acids, which help lower the risk of cardiovascular disease. A single portion of canned sardines (3.5 oz/100 g) provides the body with 2 to 3 days' worth of omega-3s.

Promote bone health
Sardines are an excellent source of vitamin D, phosphorus and calcium (if eaten with the bones), three elements that play an essential role in bone health.

Lower the risk of renal cancer
Eating oily fish at least once a week has been shown to significantly lower the risk of renal cancer.

Rejuvenate the skin
Sardines are complete proteins and help repair and maintain body tissue (skin, muscle, bone).

THINGS TO REMEMBER
• It's recommended to cook sardines in a foil packet to help preserve their omega-3 fatty acids.

• Eating canned fish, including the bones (with caution), helps increase calcium levels.

HOW TO EAT IT
Fresh: grilled, in bouillabaisse or as a tapas.

Canned: on canapés or in a salad.

DID YOU KNOW?

Small fish such as sardines contain fewer pollutants, such as mercury, than large ones, because they don't store heavy metals.

STRAWBERRIES

Composition

EXCELLENT SOURCE OF: vitamin C

GOOD SOURCE OF: manganese, fiber

SOURCE OF: folate, magnesium, potassium, vitamin B$_6$, iron

Strawberries are packed with antioxidants, including flavonoids (anthocyanins) and phenolic acids (ellagic acid).

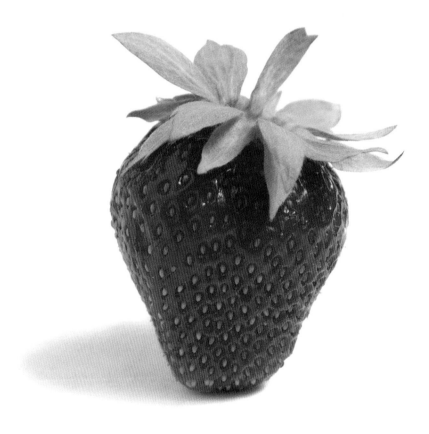

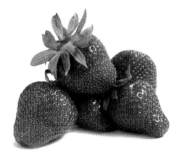

This delicious summer berry is bursting with nutrients. The Romans grew strawberries in their gardens thousands of years ago.

VIRTUES

Improve skin's elasticity
The high concentration of vitamin C found in strawberries helps produce collagen, which in turn helps prevent dry skin and wrinkles that appear with age.

Boost gray matter
The antioxidants found in strawberries keep the brain healthy and young. Incorporating strawberries into a diet has been shown to slow cognitive decline.

Protect against cardiovascular disease
The flavonoids found in strawberries help lower the risk of atherosclerosis (a condition in which plaque builds up inside arteries), which often leads to cardiovascular disease.

Boast anticancer properties
Strawberries have a high level of ellagic acid, which has been shown to prevent cancerous tumors from developing by depriving them of the oxygen and nutrients they need in order to grow and multiple.

THINGS TO REMEMBER

• Eating strawberries on a daily basis (at least 1½ cups/375 ml) has been shown to significantly increase the body's ability to create antioxidants.

• Eight strawberries contain more vitamin C than an orange.

• It's best to consume strawberries shortly after buying or picking them — this ensures you're benefitting from as much vitamin C as this power berry has to offer.

HOW TO EAT IT

• In smoothies, mousse, coulis, jams or sorbet.

• In a green salad, with shrimp and avocado.

• On a grilled fruit kabob, with chocolate fondue, in a yogurt or ricotta parfait.

-------- **QUICK STRAWBERRY JAM** --------

Want to make homemade strawberry jam in a flash? Using a fork, mash 1 cup (250 ml) of strawberries, add 3 tbsp of chia seeds and mix together. Refrigerate for 2 hours. Can be kept in the refrigerator for up to one week.

TOMATO

Composition

SOURCE OF: vitamins A, B$_6$, C, E and K, folate, copper, potassium, manganese

Tomatoes contain carotenoids, including lycopene, lutein, beta-carotene and zeaxanthin.

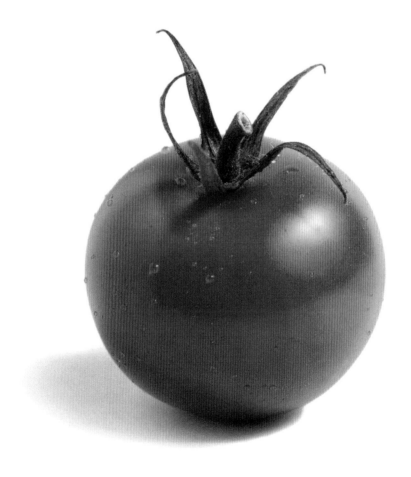

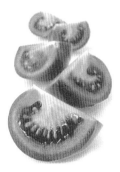

Is the tomato a fruit or a vegetable? From a strictly botanical point of view, tomatoes are considered fruit (berries, to be more precise) seeing as, contrary to vegetables, they contain the seeds of the plant. However, from a culinary perspective, tomatoes are considered vegetables (a term used to differentiate plants that are consumed as part of a savory meal from those used in sweeter dishes).

VIRTUES

Lower the risk of certain cancers
Cooked tomatoes are the best-known source of lycopene — a phytochemical that is enhanced when tomatoes are cooked. A high consumption of this powerful carotenoid could reduce the risk of prostate cancer by up to 30%. The various antioxidants found in the tomato also help lower the chances of such cancer.

Keep skin looking young
Tomato paste, rich as it is in lycopene, has the ability to neutralize free radicals caused by exposure to the sun, promote collagen production, slow down the process of aging and keep skin looking younger longer.

Improve blood cholesterol levels
A regular consumption of tomatoes or tomato-derived products (such as tomato juice, tomato sauce and tomato paste) has been shown to reduce oxidation of LDL cholesterol (the "bad" cholesterol).

Lower the risk of cardiovascular complications
The consumption of tomato extract or tomato-based products has been shown to reduce platelet aggregation, the formation of blood clots that can lead to clogged arteries.

THINGS TO REMEMBER
• Bright red tomatoes contain up to twice the amount of lycopene found in pale tomatoes. Tomatoes that are left to mature on the plant also contain more lycopene than tomatoes that have been picked green and left to ripen in the open.

• The skin of a tomato contains more antioxidants than its flesh or seeds.

• It's highly recommended to eat the skin of a tomato, as it is packed with lycopene. Lycopene is fat-soluble, therefore it is best consumed with a bit of oil for easier absorption.

• When buying canned tomato products (i.e., tomato paste), opt for those that are low in sodium.

HOW TO EAT IT
• In gazpacho or bruschetta, in a salad with mozzarella cheese, fresh basil and a drizzle of olive oil, in sandwiches.

• In soups, stuffed or as a side dish.

• Juiced, in sauces or as a paste.

WALNUTS

Composition

EXCELLENT SOURCE OF: manganese

GOOD SOURCE OF: copper, magnesium

SOURCE OF: protein, vitamins B_1, B_3 and B_6,
folate, zinc, phosphorus, iron, fiber

Walnuts are rich in omega-3 fatty acids,
phytosterols and phenolic acids
(ellagic acid and gallic acid).

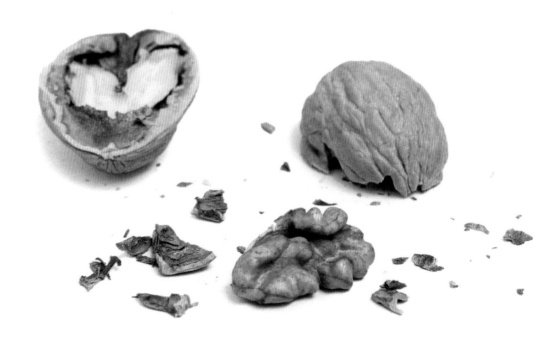

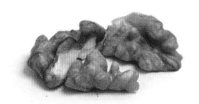

The Latin name for the walnut tree, *Juglans*, is a contraction of *Jovis* and *glans*, which means "the gland of Jupiter," referring to the Roman belief that the highly fertile walnut tree had been given to them by Jupiter.

VIRTUES

Lower cholesterol
According to several studies, a regular consumption of walnuts (5 portions of ¼ cup/ 60 ml per week) helps lower the body's total cholesterol and LDL cholesterol levels (the "bad" cholesterol) and increase HDL cholesterol levels (the "good" cholesterol).

Prevent cardiovascular disease
A regular consumption of walnuts has been shown to reduce the risk of cardiovascular disease by approximately 40%.

Improve motor and behavioral skills
Rich in antioxidants and plant-based omega-3s, walnuts promote brain health, have a positive effect on motor and behavioral skills and help boost memory.

Prevent certain cancers
Several studies claim that the phytosterols found in walnuts could have a preventative effect on breast and prostate cancers.

THINGS TO REMEMBER
Walnuts contain 70% polyunsaturated fat. Plus their omega-3 to omega-6 ratio is ideal for your health.

STORING
Walnuts are subject to oxidation and can turn rancid quickly. It's best to purchase in-shell walnuts, as their casing protects them against air and light. Store nuts in an airtight container and keep refrigerated or store in the freezer.

HOW TO EAT IT
• As a snack, roasted or raw, in a trail mix with dried fruit.

• In Waldorf or endive salad, with cereal, yogurt or in granola bars.

• As a tapenade, in stuffing, bread, pasta sauce or on cheese platters.

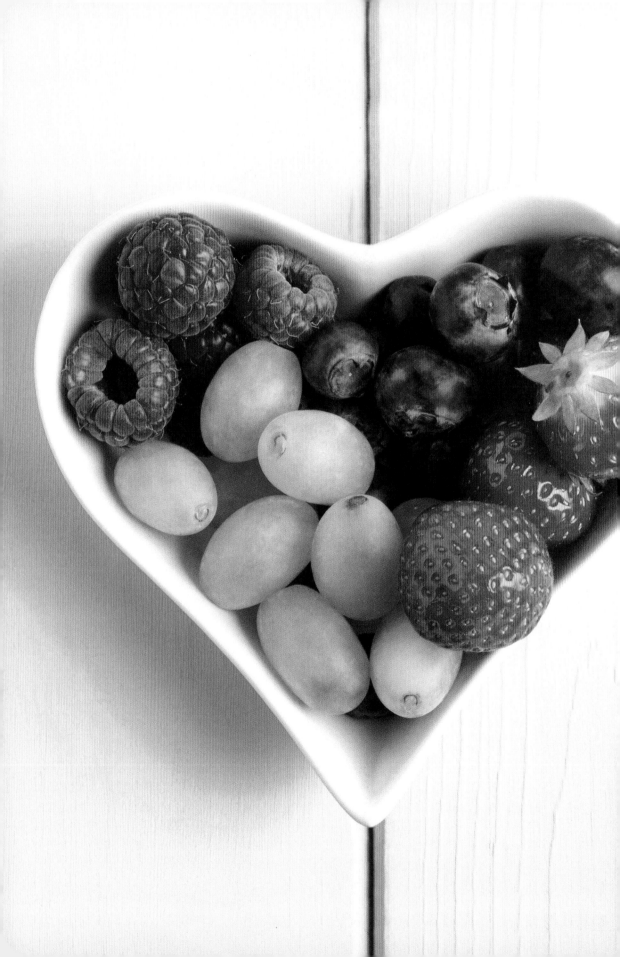

FACT OR
FICTION

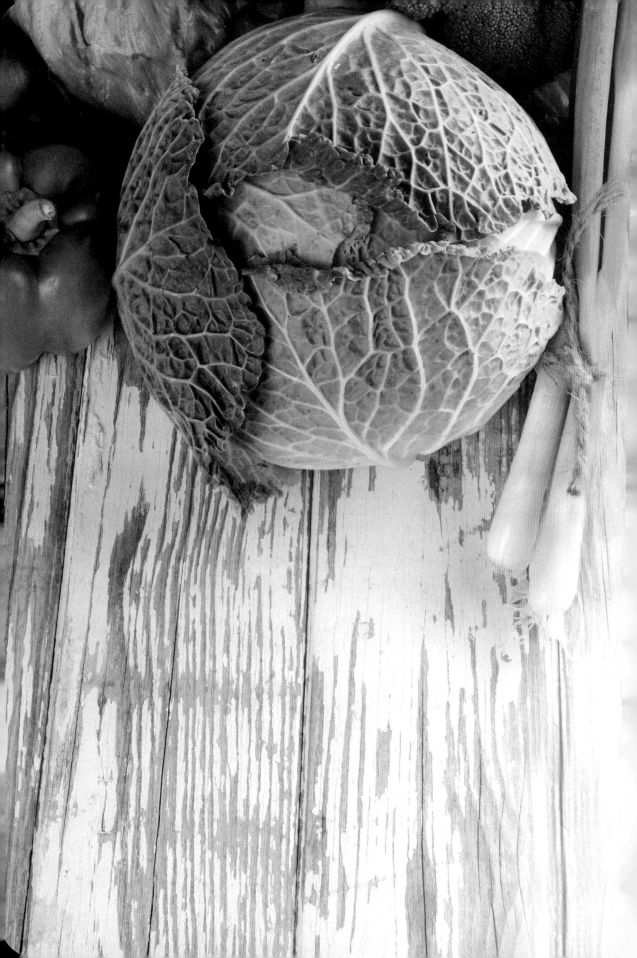

YOU SHOULD ONLY EAT ORGANIC FRUITS AND VEGETABLES.

FALSE.

According to a number of studies, organic fruits and vegetables have more antioxidants (although sometimes marginally more) than regular ones. They are not treated with pesticides or fungicides, so the plants naturally produce more of these nutrients to protect against attack.

Every year, in the United States, the Environmental Working Group studies the amount of pesticide residue in some 40 fruits and vegetables. For food with the least residue, you do not need to buy organic. But it is a good idea to choose organic products for food that does contain the most residue. (See table below.)

If you don't eat organic food, you should still eat fruits and vegetables from traditional agriculture rather than eliminating them from your diet. Pesticides are much less of a health risk than deficiencies in fiber, vitamins, minerals and phytonutrients from a diet that doesn't include many fruits and vegetables. The risk of pesticide residue is negligible compared with the health benefits of a diet with plenty of fruits and vegetables.

CLEAN 15	DIRTY DOZEN
Asparagus	Apples
Avocados	Celery
Cabbage	Cherry tomatoes
Cantaloupe	Chile peppers
Cauliflower	Cucumber
Corn	Grapes
Eggplant	Nectarines
Grapefruit	Peaches
Kiwi	Potatoes
Mango	Red peppers
Onions	Spinach
Papaya	Strawberries
Peas	
Pineapple	
Sweet potato	

FRESH VEGETABLES ARE MORE NUTRITIOUS THAN FROZEN.

FALSE.
Contrary to popular belief, fresh vegetables are not necessarily more nutritious than frozen.

Generally, the fresher the food, the more nutritious it is, because vitamins and minerals are sensitive to light, oxygen and heat. Fruits and vegetables should be eaten as soon as possible after they are picked.

Fresh vegetables: When vegetables are bought fresh from the market or the grocery store, they may have spent a long time in transport and storage and therefore lose a significant amount of nutrients.

Frozen vegetables: Fresh vegetables destined for freezing are processed a few hours after being picked. The storage time is very short, preserving their nutrients. The vegetables are blanched (dipped in boiling water) before being frozen, a process that reduces their content of water-soluble vitamins (in particular vitamins B_1 and C) and certain antioxidants. However, other nutrients (such as water-soluble vitamins A and E) are better preserved, so frozen vegetables contain more than fresh vegetables.

Whether fresh or frozen, all vegetables are good sources of nutrients and fiber. Variety is the healthiest bet.

PRE-CUT VEGETABLES AREN'T NUTRITIOUS.

FALSE.
Luckily for busy people, the vitamin and mineral content of pre-cut vegetables is still pretty good. Of course, they are less rich in vitamin C and folate than whole fresh vegetables, but still a considerable amount remains. For example, women need 75 mg of vitamin C per day. Even if the content of vitamin C in a green pepper is reduced 20% when it is pre-cut, it will still meet 95% of her needs. Plus, it won't be the only source of vitamin C during the day.

So don't be afraid to make life easier for yourself. The important thing with vegetables is to eat them.

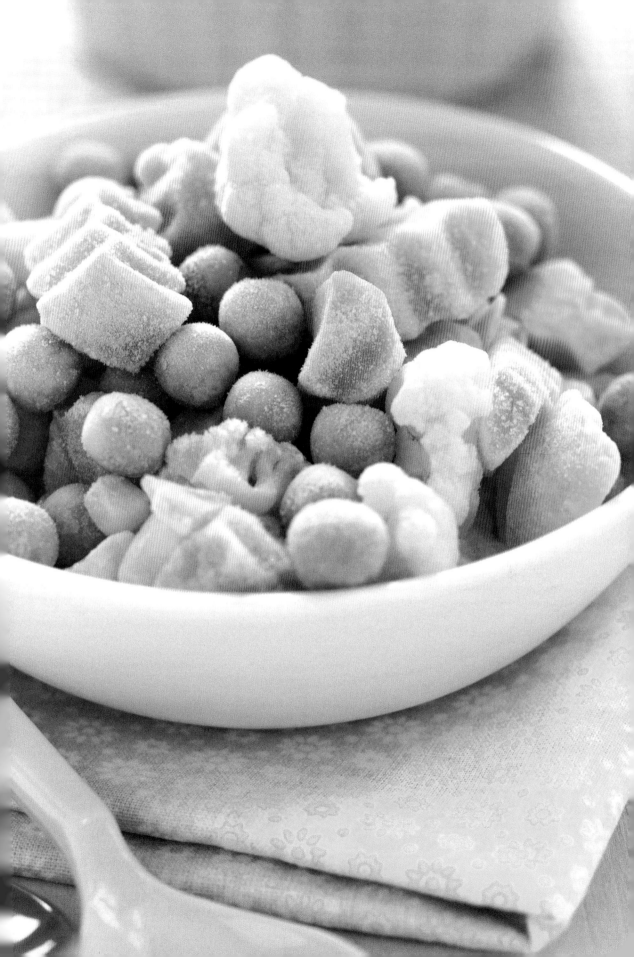

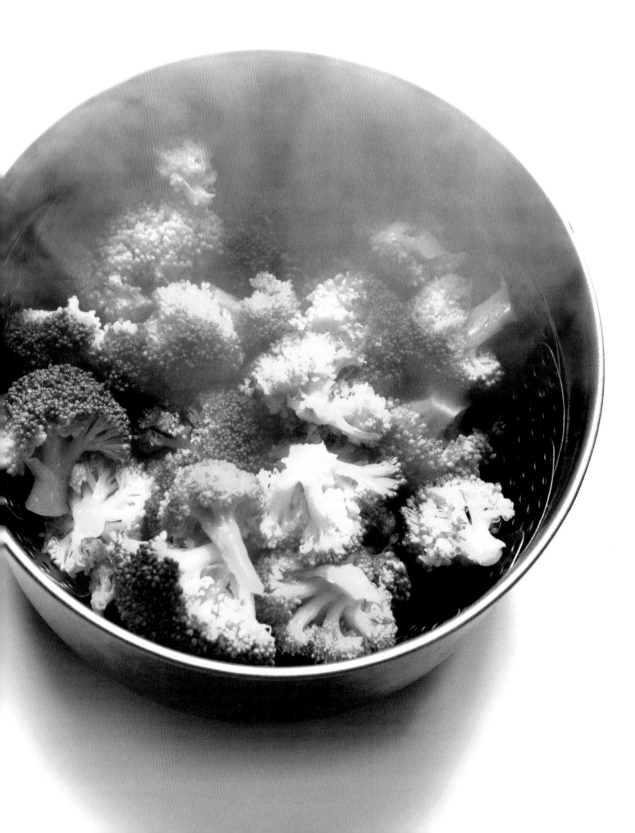

COOKING REDUCES THE NUTRITIONAL VALUE OF FOOD.

FALSE, HOWEVER . . .

Overcooking can cause foods to lose some of their vitamins, especially when cooked in water, as the water will absorb most of the food's minerals. It's recommended to cook and serve vegetables as quickly as possible. The best cooking methods for preserving a food's nutrients are sautéing, steaming and roasting. However, some foods, like orange vegetables (carrots, sweet potatoes, etc.) and tomatoes, actually contain more anti-oxidants when cooked. For example, according to some studies, the amount of lycopene (an antioxidant) in a tomato doubles after 30 minutes of cooking time. And finally, it's important to remember that cooking helps destroy unwanted bacteria and helps with digestion.

While it's true that raw veggies contain more vitamins and help with weight control (they make you feel fuller), the key to a balanced diet is variety — so make sure to eat your share of both cooked and raw vegetables.

MICROWAVING VEGETABLES DESTROYS THEIR NUTRIENTS.

FALSE.

Studies back it up — microwaving and steaming are the best ways to preserve a vegetable's healthy nutrients. Remember: quickly cook your veggies and avoid letting them come in contact with the cooking water.

RIPE FRUITS AND VEGETABLES ARE BETTER FOR YOU.

TRUE.

Generally speaking, fruits and vegetables contain more nutritional elements when they're fully mature. There are a few exceptions. Take, for example, broccoli sprouts — they contain more antioxidants than mature broccoli. As a rule, however, fruits and vegetables become richer in vitamins and minerals the more they mature, with a lot of their nutritional benefits coming from the pigments that give them their color. Of course, other factors (sun, heat, soil, etc.) can also influence how many nutrients a food ends up with. Taste-wise, it goes without saying that fruits and vegetables are at their peak when they're left to ripen to perfection.

TIPS FOR PRESERVING VITAMINS AND MINERALS

- Eat fruits and vegetables soon after buying or picking them. The longer they are stored, the more nutrients they lose.

- Wash whole vegetables and don't let them soak, to limit the loss of water-soluble vitamins (see table below).

- Preferably, don't cut fruits and vegetables too much in advance because many vitamins are sensitive to oxygen and light.

- Limit cooking time for vegetables (serve them crunchy) to preserve heat-sensitive nutrients. Exceptions: lycopene, found in tomatoes, and quercetin, found in onions. These two antioxidants are not broken down by heat; in fact they are more easily assimilated after cooking.

- Ideally, steam vegetables to prevent water-soluble vitamins from leaching into the cooking water.

- To preserve fat-soluble vitamins (see table below), which are not highly water soluble, braise, steam or boil.

- When cooking in water, bring the water to a boil and then add the vegetables (except for potatoes, which are added to cold water).

- Avoid frying or cooking at high temperatures, because this produces potentially carcinogenic, toxic compounds.

WATER-SOLUBLE VITAMINS	FAT-SOLUBLE VITAMINS
B complex vitamins	Vitamin A
Vitamin C	Vitamin D
	Vitamin E
	Vitamin K

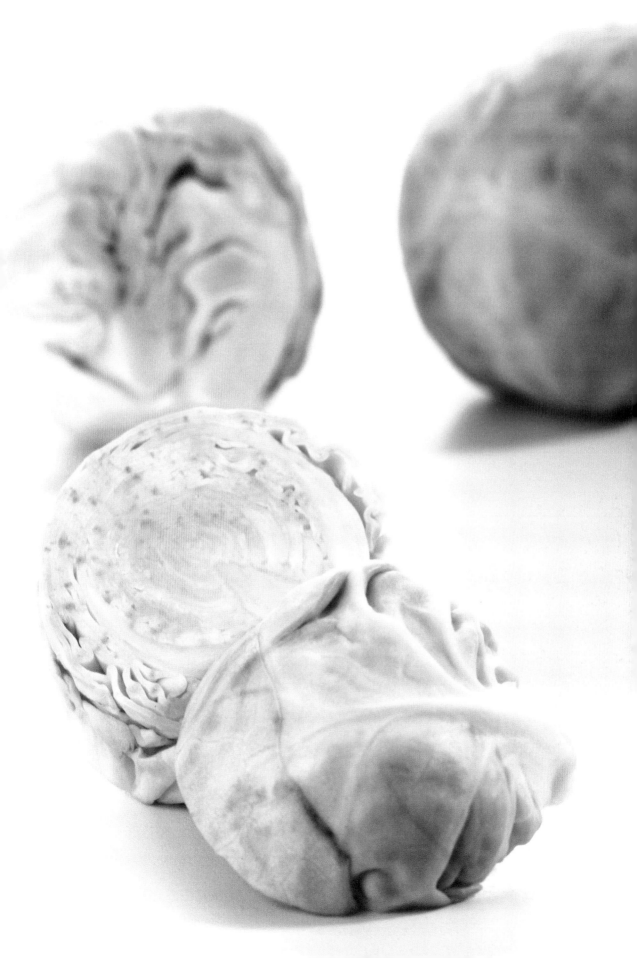

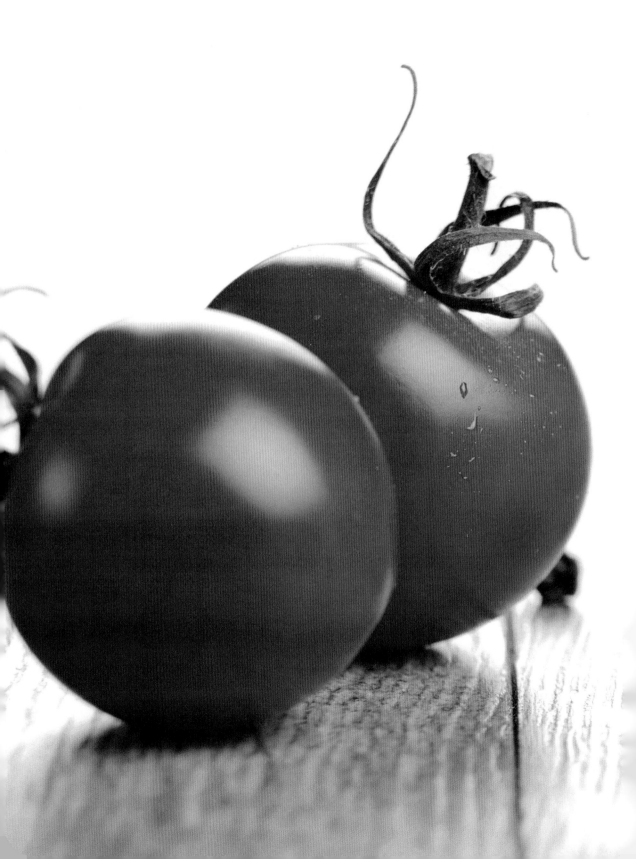

RECESIPES

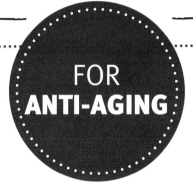

FOR
ANTI-AGING

LEGEND

🥣 Preparation   ❄️ Refrigeration

🫙 Marinating   🌡️ Freezing

🥄 Soaking   🍲 Cooking

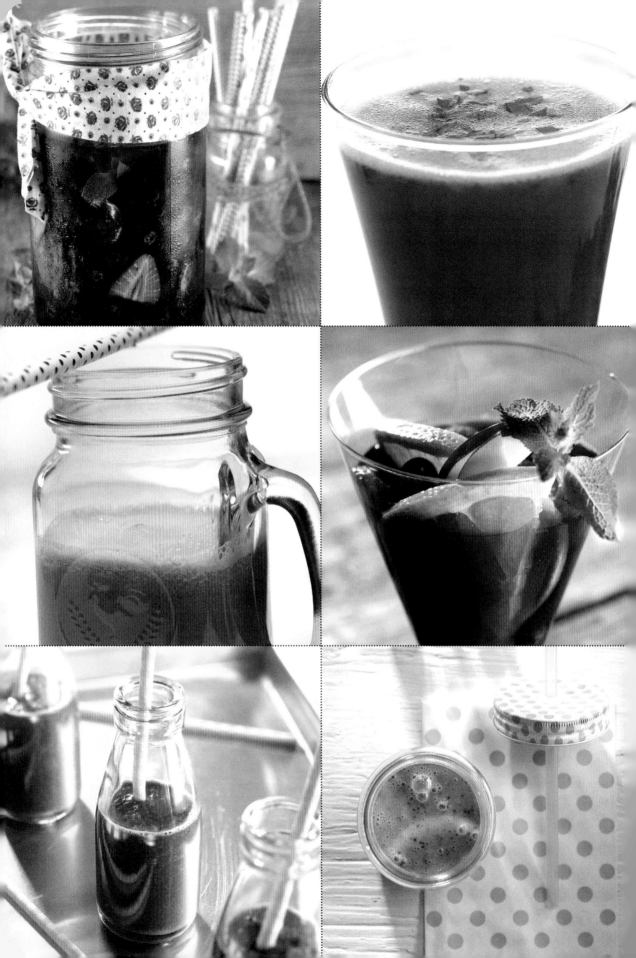

DRINKS

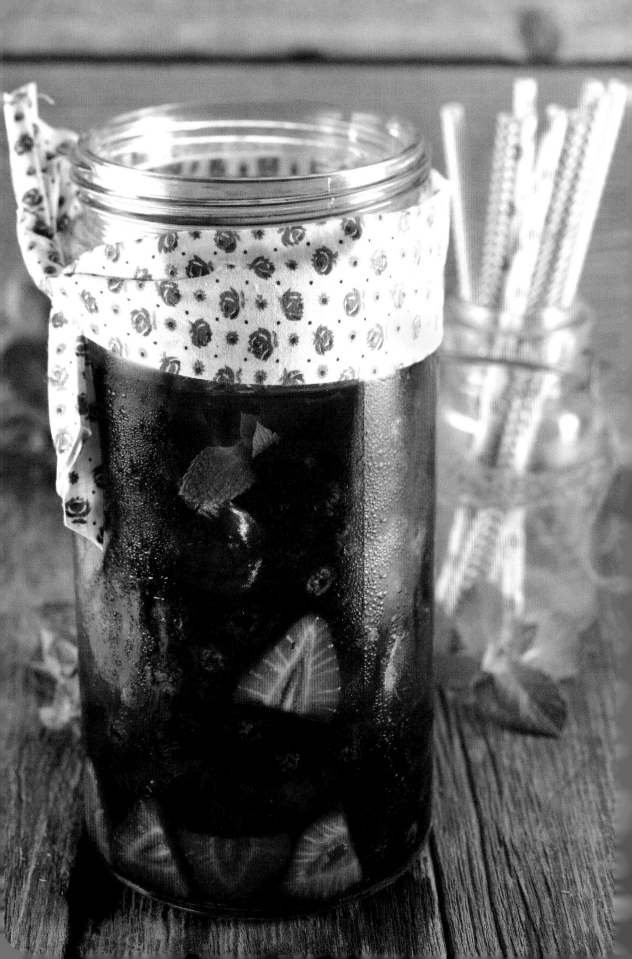

FRUIT-INFUSED
— ICED TEA —

4 SERVINGS
5 MINUTES

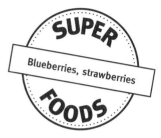
SUPER FOODS
Blueberries, strawberries

INGREDIENTS

2 cups (500 ml) green tea

2 cups (500 ml) frozen **blueberries**

16 large **strawberries**, sliced

Cubed or crushed ice

4 fresh mint leaves

METHOD

In a pitcher, carefully stir together tea, blueberries, strawberries and ice.

Serve in glasses and garnish with mint leaves.

Nutrition Facts Per serving	
Amount	% Daily Value
Calories 50	
Fat 0.5 g	1%
Saturated 0 g	
+ Trans 0 g	
Polyunsaturated 0 g	
Omega-6 0 g	
Omega-3 0 g	
Monounsaturated 0 g	
Cholesterol 0 mg	0%
Sodium 5 mg	0%
Potassium 85 mg	2%
Carbohydrates 12 g	4%
Fiber 3 g	12%
Sugar 8 g	
Protein 0.4 g	
Vitamin A 10 ER	2%
Vitamin C 2 mg	4%
Calcium 7 mg	0%
Iron 0.2 mg	2%
Phosphorus 9.2 mg	0%

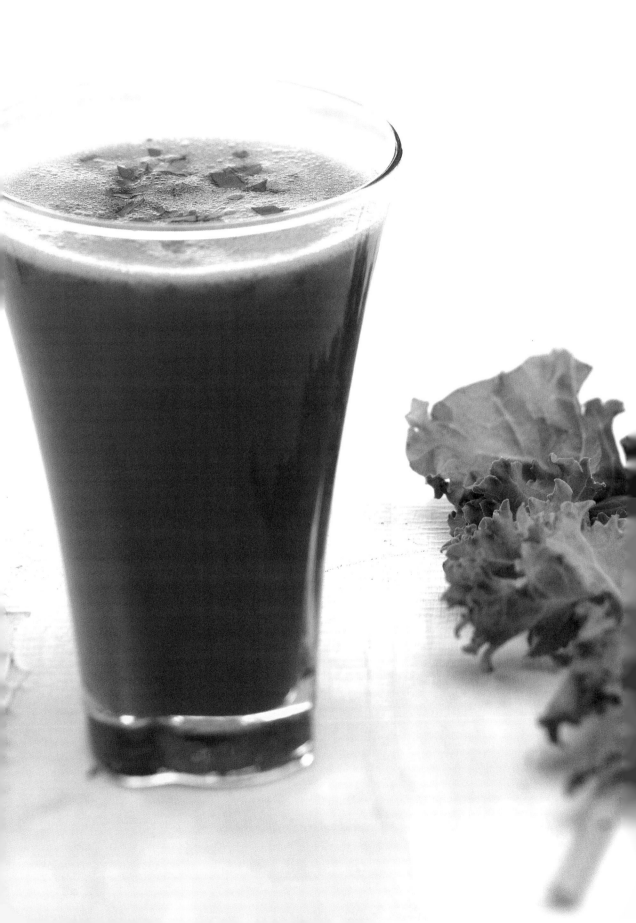

GREEN JUICE
WITH KALE

2 SERVINGS
5 MINUTES

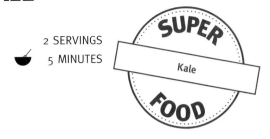

SUPER
Kale
FOOD

INGREDIENTS

8 **kale** leaves

1 cucumber

4 stalks celery

2 green apples

2 fresh mint leaves

1 tbsp chopped fresh cilantro

Juice of 1 lemon

1 tsp minced fresh ginger

METHOD

In a juicer, juice kale, cucumber, celery, apples, mint and cilantro.

Add lemon juice and ginger. Mix well.

Nutrition Facts Per serving	
Amount	**% Daily Value**
Calories 130	
Fat 1 g	2%
Saturated 0.1 g	
+ Trans 0 g	
Polyunsaturated 0.3 g	
Omega-6 0.2 g	
Omega-3 0.1 g	
Monounsaturated 0.1 g	
Cholesterol 0 mg	0%
Sodium 115 mg	5%
Potassium 730 mg	21%
Carbohydrates 28 g	9%
Fiber 7 g	28%
Sugar 18 g	
Protein 3 g	
Vitamin A 341 ER	35%
Vitamin C 35 mg	60%
Calcium 142 mg	15%
Iron 1.2 mg	8%
Phosphorus 76.4 mg	6%

GRAPEFRUIT
ELIXIR

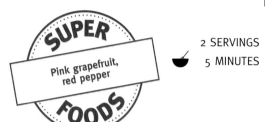

2 SERVINGS

5 MINUTES

INGREDIENTS

1 **pink grapefruit**, peeled

1 **red pepper**

3 carrots

1 apple

Juice of 1 lemon

METHOD

In a juicer, juice grapefruit, red pepper, carrot and apple.

Add lemon juice and stir.

Nutrition Facts Per serving	
Amount	**% Daily Value**
Calories 100	
Fat 0.5 g	1%
Saturated 0.1 g + Trans 0 g	
Polyunsaturated 0.2 g	
Omega-6 0.2 g	
Omega-3 0 g	
Monounsaturated 0 g	
Cholesterol 0 mg	0%
Sodium 85 mg	4%
Potassium 570 mg	16%
Carbohydrates 22 g	7%
Fiber 5 g	20%
Sugar 12 g	
Protein 2 g	
Vitamin A 1656 ER	170%
Vitamin C 103 mg	170%
Calcium 59 mg	6%
Iron 0.6 mg	4%
Phosphorus 65.7 mg	6%

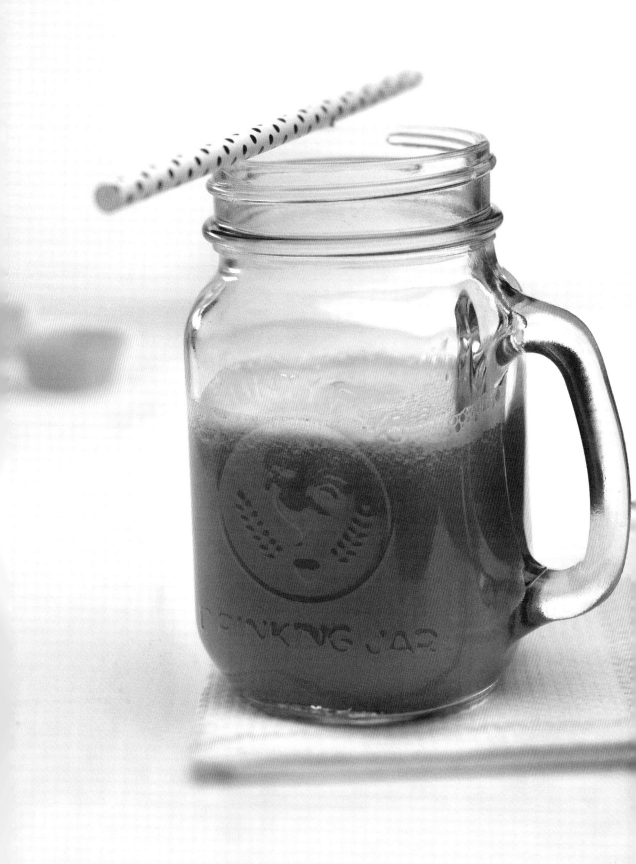

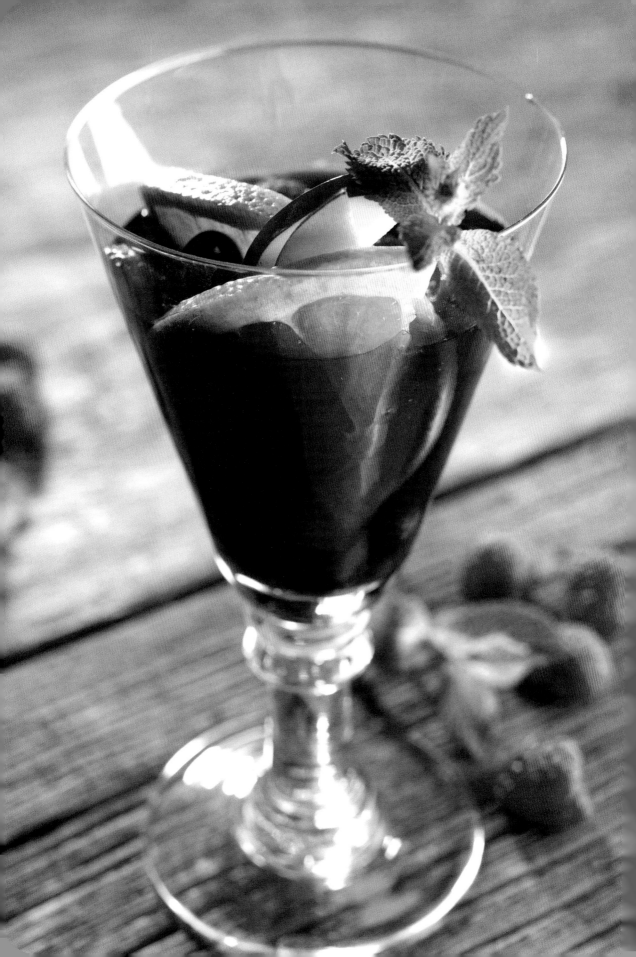

REJUVENATING
SANGRIA

8 SERVINGS
10 MINUTES

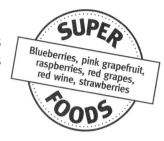

Blueberries, pink grapefruit, raspberries, red grapes, red wine, strawberries

INGREDIENTS

1 bottle (750 ml) **red wine**

2 cups (500 ml) sparkling lemon water

2 cups (500 ml) **red grape** juice

1 orange, sliced

1 **pink grapefruit**, sliced

1 apple, sliced

10 **strawberries**, sliced

½ cup (125 ml) frozen **blueberries**

½ cup (125 ml) frozen **raspberries**

Handful of fresh mint leaves

METHOD

In a large pitcher, combine wine, lemon water and grape juice. Add orange, grapefruit, apple and strawberries. Stir.

Just before serving, add blueberries and raspberries.

Garnish with mint leaves.

Nutrition Facts Per serving	
Amount	% Daily Value
Calories 100	
Fat 0.1 g	0%
Saturated 0 g	
+ Trans 0 g	
Polyunsaturated 0 g	
Omega-6 0 g	
Omega-3 0 g	
Monounsaturated 0 g	
Cholesterol 0 mg	0%
Sodium 15 mg	1%
Potassium 190 mg	5%
Carbohydrates 25 g	8%
Fiber 2 g	8%
Sugar 20 g	
Protein 1 g	
Vitamin A 33 ER	4%
Vitamin C 22 mg	35%
Calcium 33 mg	4%
Iron 0.8 mg	6%
Phosphorus 22.4 mg	2%

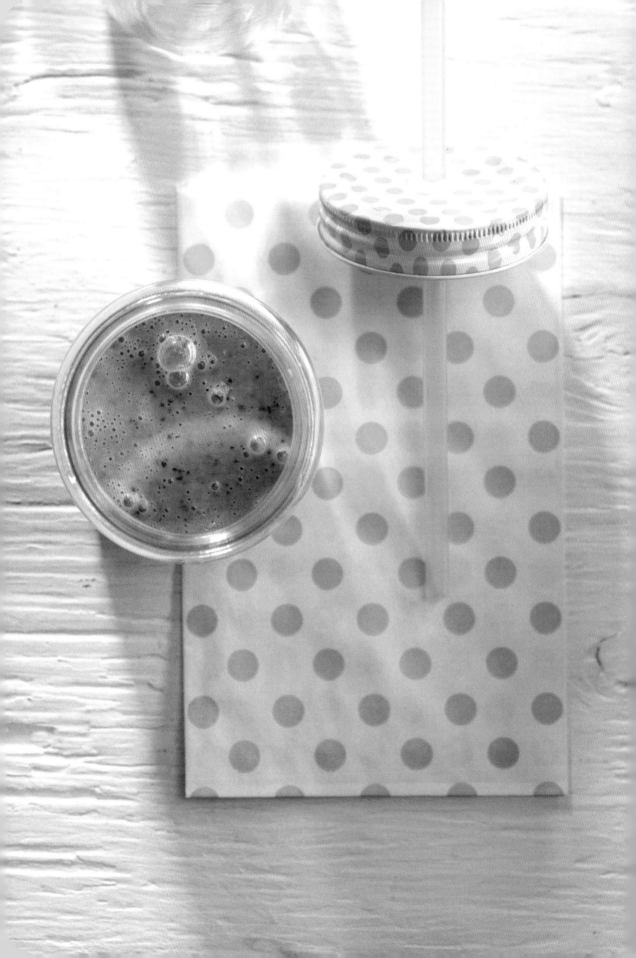

BLUEBERRY AND POMEGRANATE
SMOOTHIE

2 SERVINGS
5 MINUTES

SUPER
Blueberries
FOOD

INGREDIENTS

½ cup (125 ml) store-bought pomegranate juice

1 cup (250 ml) regular or almond milk

¼ cup (60 ml) plain Greek yogurt

¾ cup (180 ml) **blueberries**

Zest of 1 lemon

Juice of ½ lemon

Ice

METHOD

In a blender, blend all the ingredients except ice for 25 to 30 seconds or until desired consistency.

Add ice and blend until smooth.

Nutrition Facts Per serving	
Amount	% Daily Value
Calories 180	
Fat 3 g	5%
Saturated 1.5 g	
+ Trans 0.1 g	
Polyunsaturated 0.2 g	
Omega-6 0.2 g	
Omega-3 0.1 g	
Monounsaturated 0.5 g	
Cholesterol 10 mg	3%
Sodium 75 mg	3%
Potassium 310 mg	9%
Carbohydrates 28 g	9%
Fiber 4 g	16%
Sugar 19 g	
Protein 9 g	
Vitamin A 76 ER	8%
Vitamin C 48 mg	80%
Calcium 226 mg	20%
Iron 1.1 mg	8%
Phosphorus 135.9 mg	10%

TOMATO AND KALE
SMOOTHIE

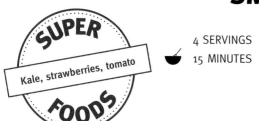

SUPER
Kale, strawberries, tomato
FOODS

🥣 4 SERVINGS
15 MINUTES

INGREDIENTS

1½ cups (375 ml) **tomato** juice

1 cup (250 ml) chopped Romaine lettuce

½ cup (125 ml) chopped fresh Italian parsley

4 **kale** leaves, coarsely chopped, stems removed

3 stalks celery, sliced

2 cucumbers, diced

2 cups (500 ml) whole **strawberries**

Juice of 1 lemon

2 tbsp chopped fresh cilantro

1 tsp minced fresh ginger

Seasoning to taste

METHOD

In a blender or food processor, combine all ingredients and blend for 25 to 30 seconds or until desired consistency.

Tip: For a richer consistency, add 1 peeled and pitted avocado.

Nutrition Facts Per serving	
Amount	**% Daily Value**
Calories 90	
Fat 1 g	2%
Saturated 0.1 g	
+ Trans 0 g	
Polyunsaturated 0.3 g	
Omega-6 0.2 g	
Omega-3 0.1 g	
Monounsaturated 0.1 g	
Cholesterol 0 mg	0%
Sodium 320 mg	14%
Potassium 810 mg	23%
Carbohydrates 18 g	6%
Fiber 5 g	20%
Sugar 10 g	
Protein 3 g	
Vitamin A 363 ER	35%
Vitamin C 90 mg	150%
Calcium 117 mg	10%
Iron 2.1 mg	15%
Phosphorus 88 mg	8%

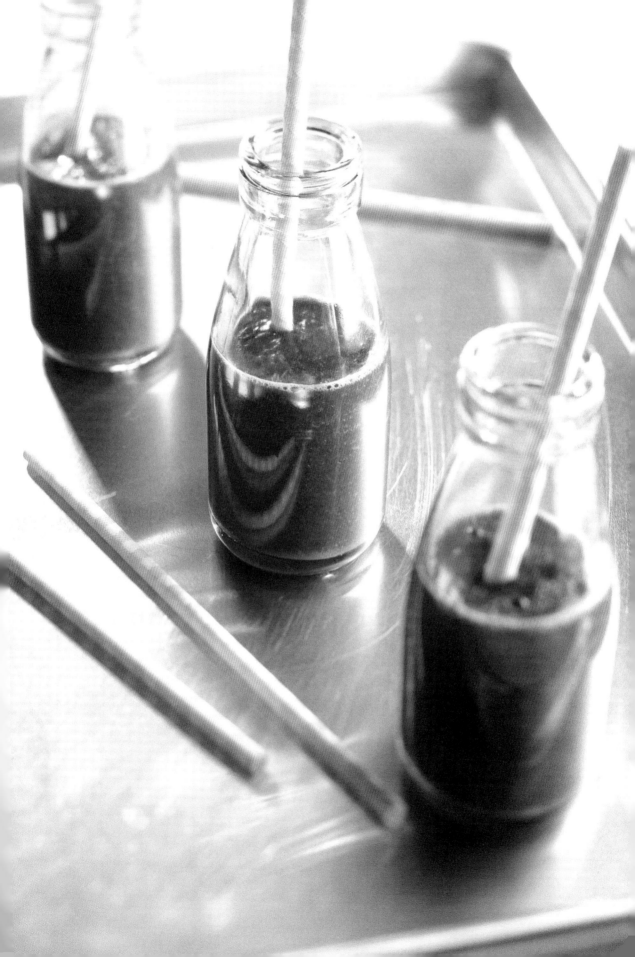

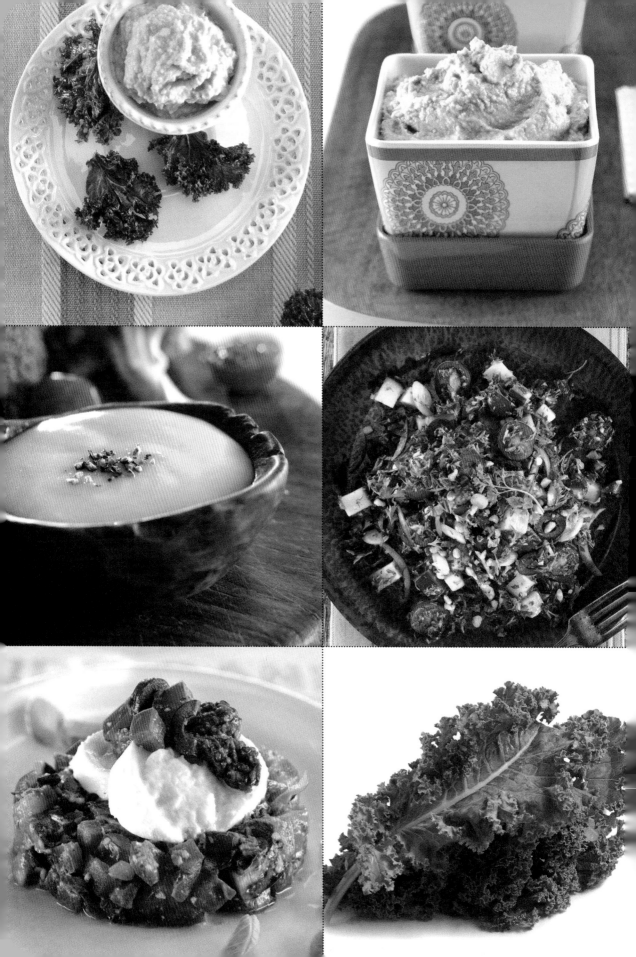

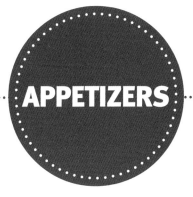

APPETIZERS

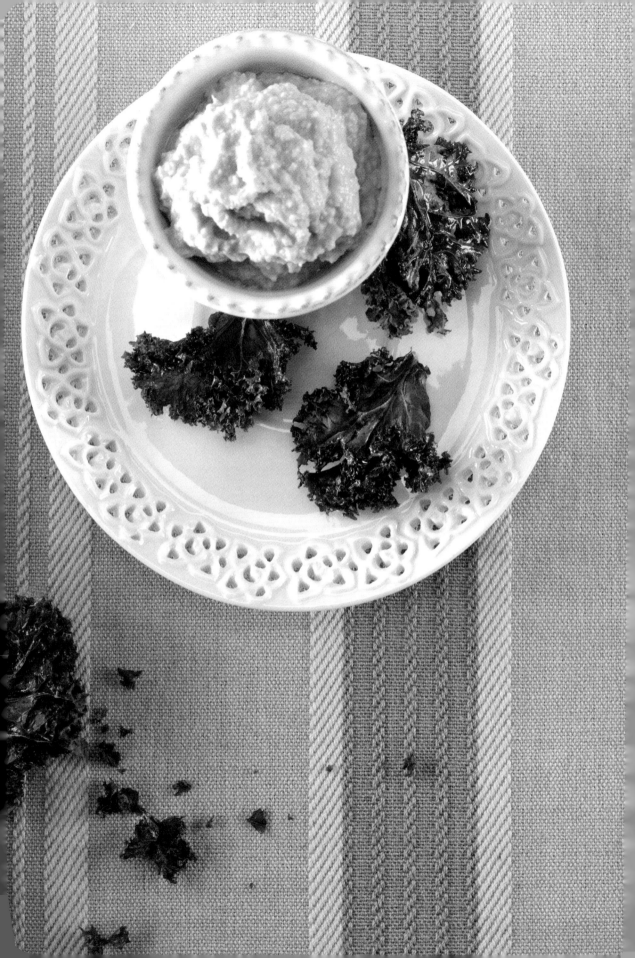

KALE
CHIPS

4 SERVINGS
10 MINUTES
15 MINUTES

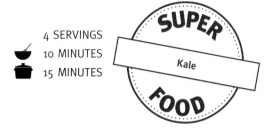

SUPER
Kale
FOOD

INGREDIENTS

10 to 12 **kale** leaves, washed and thoroughly dried

2 tbsp olive oil

Juice of 1 lime

Seasoning to taste

METHOD

Position rack in center of oven and preheat to 350°F (180°C). Line a baking sheet with parchment paper.

Remove stems from kale leaves. Tear into bite-sized pieces.

In a large bowl, combine olive oil and lime juice. Coat kale leaves evenly and season to taste. Place kale on prepared baking sheet.

Bake in center of preheated oven, turning partway through cooking, about 15 minutes or until leaves are crisp but still green. Keep a close eye on the chips so as not to burn them.

Serve with Edamame Purée (see recipe p. 86) or Lima Bean and Caramelized Onion Purée (see recipe p. 170).

Nutrition Facts Per serving	
Amount	**% Daily Value**
Calories 80	
Fat 7 g	11%
Saturated 1 g + Trans 0 g	
Polyunsaturated 0.5 g	
Omega-6 0.5 g	
Omega-3 0.1 g	
Monounsaturated 5 g	
Cholesterol 0 mg	0%
Sodium 5 mg	0%
Potassium 50 mg	1%
Carbohydrates 2 g	1%
Fiber 1 g	4%
Sugar 0 g	
Protein 1 g	
Vitamin A 190 ER	20%
Vitamin C 11 mg	20%
Calcium 42 mg	4%
Iron 0.1 mg	0%
Phosphorus 3.2 mg	0%

EDAMAME
PURÉE

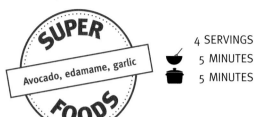

SUPER FOODS

Avocado, edamame, garlic

4 SERVINGS
5 MINUTES
5 MINUTES

INGREDIENTS

2 cups (500 ml) frozen **edamame**, shelled

⅓ cup (80 ml) water

1 ripe **avocado**, diced

Juice of 1 lemon

2 tbsp tahini (sesame butter)

1 clove **garlic**, minced

1 tbsp minced fresh ginger

Seasoning to taste

METHOD

In a saucepan of boiling water, cook edamame for 3 minutes.

In a food processor, purée all ingredients until well blended. Adjust seasoning.

Serve with crackers or raw veggies.

Nutrition Facts Per serving	
Amount	**% Daily Value**
Calories 310	
Fat 18 g	28%
Saturated 3 g	
+ Trans 0 g	
Polyunsaturated 2.5 g	
Omega-6 2.5 g	
Omega-3 0.1 g	
Monounsaturated 6 g	
Cholesterol 0 mg	0%
Sodium 390 mg	16%
Potassium 310 mg	9%
Carbohydrates 18 g	6%
Fiber 10 g	40%
Sugar 2 g	
Protein 18 g	
Vitamin A 38 ER	4%
Vitamin C 16 mg	25%
Calcium 139 mg	15%
Iron 3.6 mg	25%
Phosphorus 93.1 mg	8%

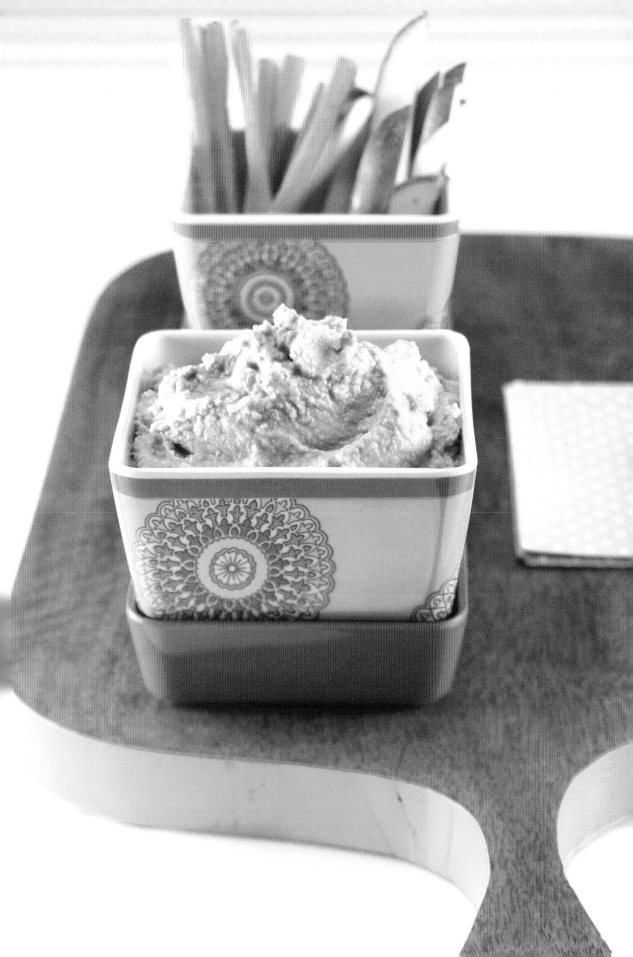

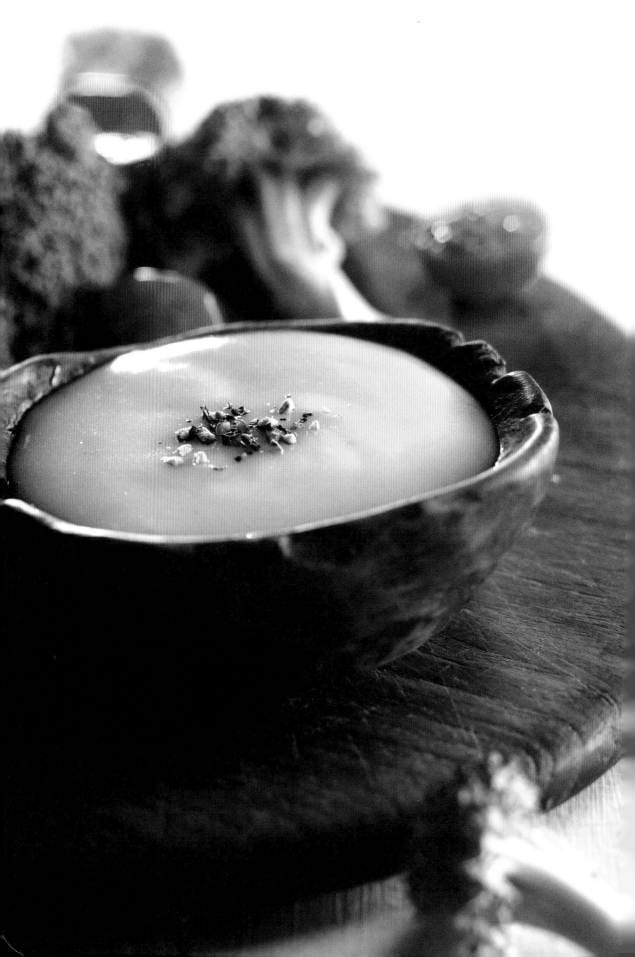

AÏOLI

16 SERVINGS OF 1 TBSP

10 MINUTES

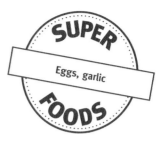

SUPER FOODS

Eggs, garlic

INGREDIENTS

5 cloves **garlic**, crushed

1 **egg** yolk

1 tbsp Dijon mustard

3 tsp lemon juice

1 cup (250 ml) olive oil

Seasoning to taste

METHOD

In a bowl, whisk together garlic, egg yolk, mustard and lemon juice.

Whisking constantly, slowly add olive oil.

Season to taste.

Serve with raw veggies (e.g., broccoli and tomatoes).

COMMON MISCONCEPTIONS

Eating garlic gives you bad breath.

TRUE, but you can easily eliminate bad breath by chomping on some parsley or mint leaves, or chewing a few coffee beans. Unfortunately, brushing your teeth won't entirely make the problem go away, as that garlicky odor doesn't just come from your mouth, but from your digestive tract as well.

Nutrition Facts Per serving	
Amount	% Daily Value
Calories 140	
Fat 14 g	22%
Saturated 2 g	
+ Trans 0 g	
Polyunsaturated 1.5 g	
Omega-6 1.5 g	
Omega-3 0.1 g	
Monounsaturated 10 g	
Cholesterol 15 mg	5%
Sodium 15 mg	1%
Potassium 35 mg	1%
Carbohydrates 3 g	1%
Fiber 0 g	0%
Sugar 0 g	
Protein 1 g	
Vitamin A 4 ER	0%
Vitamin C 4 mg	6%
Calcium 16 mg	2%
Iron 0.3 mg	2%
Phosphorus 16.1 mg	2%

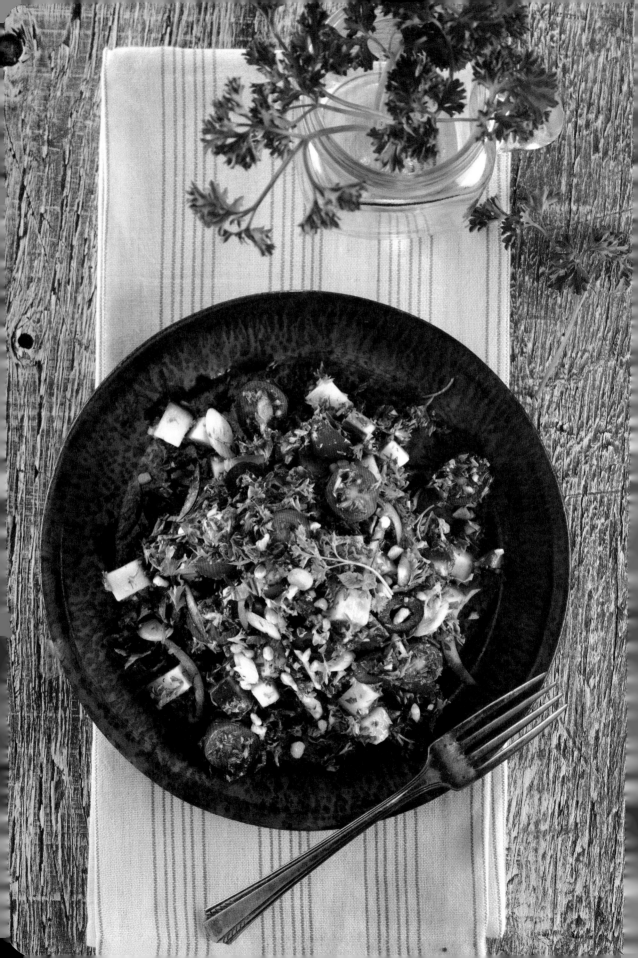

KALE
TABBOULEH

6 SERVINGS
20 MINUTES

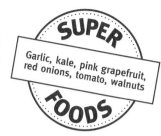

SUPER FOODS

Garlic, kale, pink grapefruit, red onions, tomato, walnuts

INGREDIENTS

2 bunches parsley, chopped

1 cup (250 ml) chopped **kale**, stems removed

½ cup (125 ml) chopped fresh mint leaves

1 cup (250 ml) cherry **tomatoes**, cut in half or quarters

1 cucumber, seeded and diced

1 small **red onion**, minced

2 tbsp chopped **walnuts**

For the vinaigrette

⅔ cup (160 ml) olive oil

½ cup (125 ml) lemon juice

¼ cup (60 ml) **grapefruit** juice

3 cloves **garlic**, minced

1 green onion, finely sliced

½ cup (125 ml) sliced pitted black olives

¼ cup (60 ml) chopped fresh mint leaves

Seasoning to taste

METHOD

In a large bowl, mix all ingredients for salad.

In a smaller bowl, whisk together ingredients for vinaigrette.

Pour vinaigrette over salad and toss to coat.

Nutrition Facts Per serving	
Amount	% Daily Value
Calories 310	
Fat 26 g	40%
Saturated 3.5 g	
+ Trans 0 g	
Polyunsaturated 1 g	
Omega-6 1 g	
Omega-3 0.2 g	
Monounsaturated 1 g	
Cholesterol 0 mg	0%
Sodium 115 mg	5%
Potassium 310 mg	9%
Carbohydrates 15 g	5%
Fiber 3 g	12%
Sugar 4 g	
Protein 3 g	
Vitamin A 255 ER	25%
Vitamin C 35 mg	60%
Calcium 100 mg	10%
Iron 1.8 mg	15%
Phosphorus 63.6 mg	6%

TOMATO, MOZZARELLA
AND PESTO TARTARE

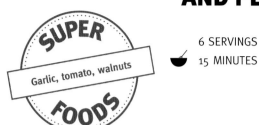

SUPER
Garlic, tomato, walnuts
FOODS

🥣 6 SERVINGS
15 MINUTES

INGREDIENTS

6 Italian **tomatoes**, diced

¼ cup (60 ml) chopped pitted black olives

1 ball (8 oz/250 g) mozzarella cheese, cut in slices

6 fresh basil leaves

For pesto

2 tbsp olive oil

1 tbsp balsamic vinegar

1 clove **garlic**, minced

½ cup (125 ml) fresh basil leaves

¼ cup (60 ml) **walnuts**

Seasoning to taste

METHOD

In a blender, blend all ingredients to make the pesto.

In a bowl, combine tomatoes and olives with half the pesto mixture.

Using a 3-inch (8 cm) round cookie cutter, arrange tomato tartare on plates. Cover with mozzarella, garnish with remaining pesto and basil leaves.

Nutrition Facts Per serving	
Amount	**% Daily Value**
Calories 230	
Fat 17 g	26%
Saturated 6 g	
+ Trans 0.2 g	
Polyunsaturated 2.5 g	
Omega-6 2 g	
Omega-3 0.5 g	
Monounsaturated 1 g	
Cholesterol 25 mg	8%
Sodium 350 mg	15%
Potassium 200 mg	6%
Carbohydrates 7 g	2%
Fiber 2 g	8%
Sugar 3 g	
Protein 12 g	
Vitamin A 162 ER	15%
Vitamin C 10 mg	15%
Calcium 317 mg	30%
Iron 0.8 mg	6%
Phosphorus 41 mg	4%

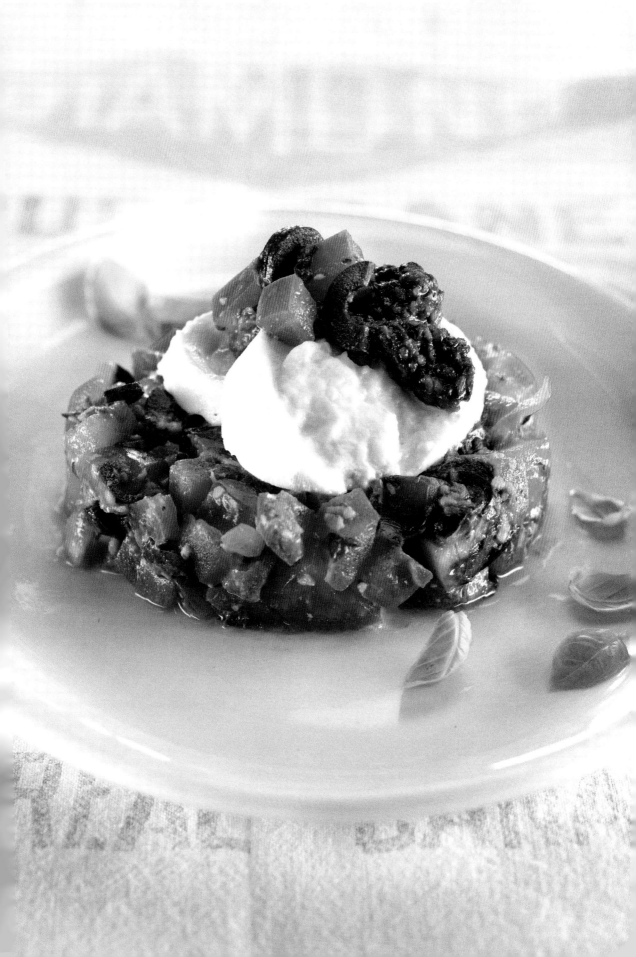

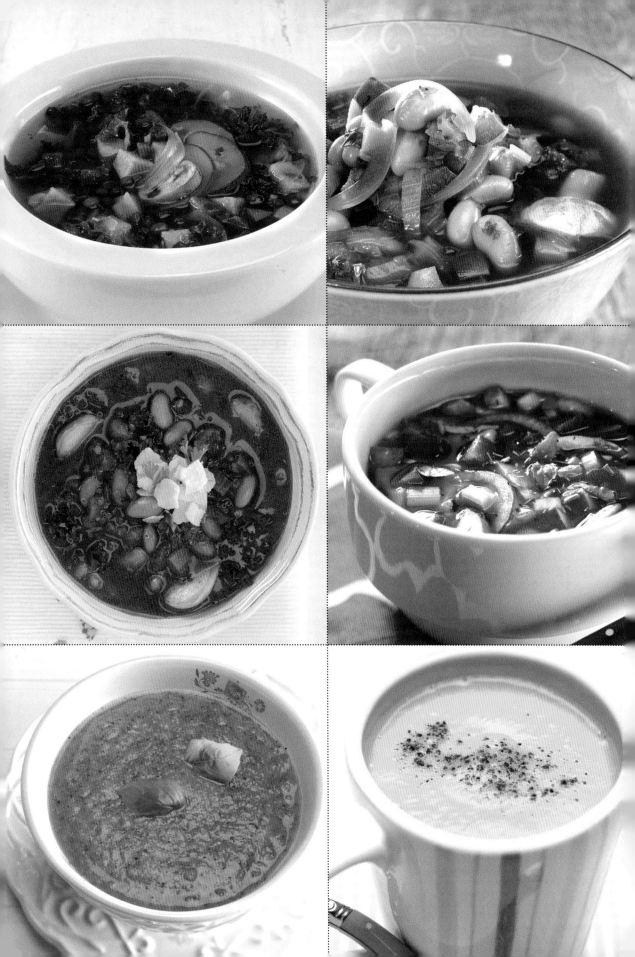

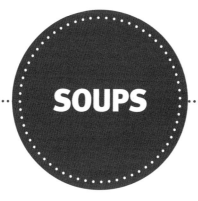

SOUPS

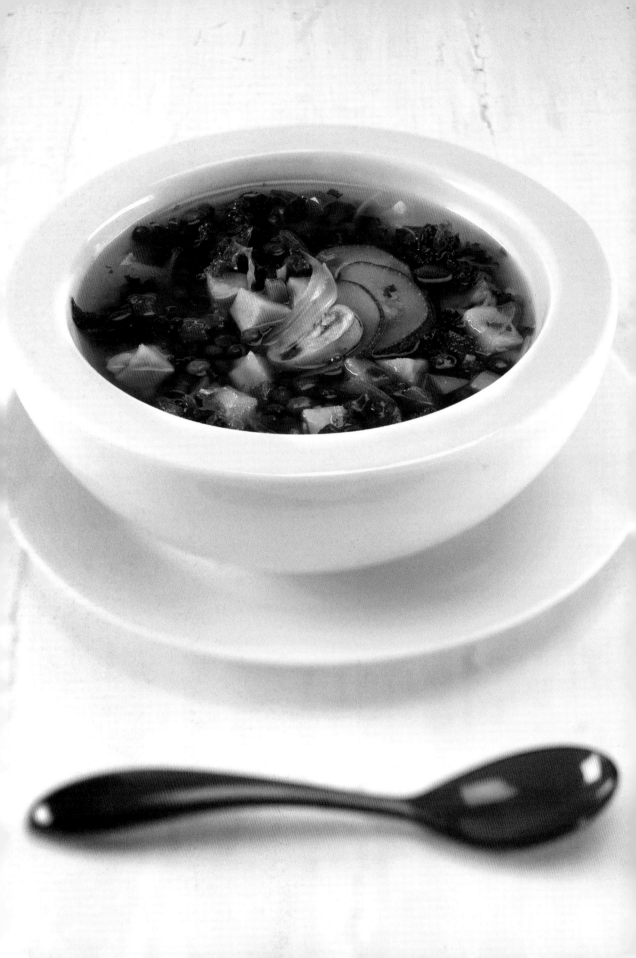

LENTIL AND
KALE SOUP

4 SERVINGS
20 MINUTES
30 MINUTES

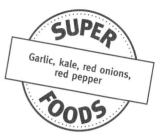

Garlic, kale, red onions, red pepper

INGREDIENTS

6 cups (1.5 liters) chicken or vegetable broth

2 cups (500 ml) chopped **kale**, stems removed

2 carrots, diced

2 zucchini, sliced

1 sweet potato, diced

1 **red pepper**, diced

2 cups (500 ml) sliced mushrooms

1 small **red onion**, minced

8 cloves **garlic**, minced

1 can (19 oz/540 ml) green lentils, drained and rinsed

Seasoning to taste

METHOD

In a large saucepan over medium heat, bring broth, kale, carrots, zucchini, sweet potato, red pepper, mushrooms, onion and garlic to a boil.

Reduce heat to low. Cover and let simmer, stirring occasionally, for 20 minutes.

Add lentils and continue cooking for 5 minutes.

Season to taste. Add water to obtain desired consistency.

Nutrition Facts Per serving	
Amount	**% Daily Value**
Calories 360	
Fat 1.5 g	2%
Saturated 0.3 g	
+ Trans 0 g	
Polyunsaturated 0.5 g	
Omega-6 0.5 g	
Omega-3 0.2 g	
Monounsaturated 0.1 g	
Cholesterol 0 mg	0%
Sodium 180 mg	8%
Potassium 1830 mg	52%
Carbohydrates 65 g	22%
Fiber 12 g	48%
Sugar 14 g	
Protein 22 g	
Vitamin A 1270 ER	130%
Vitamin C 98 mg	160%
Calcium 217 mg	20%
Iron 5.9 mg	40%
Phosphorus 428.5 mg	40%

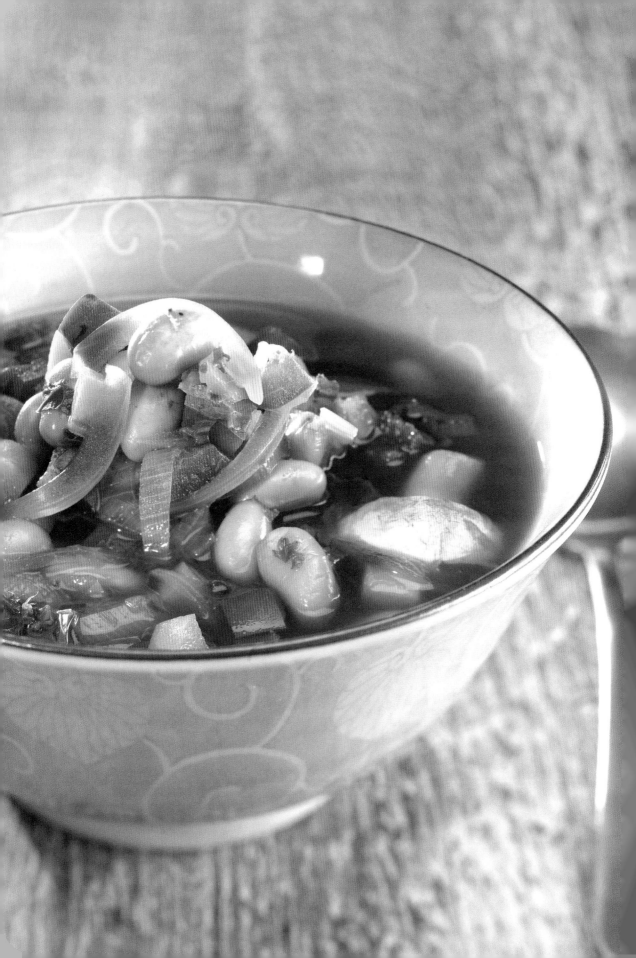

EDAMAME
SOUP

4 TO 6 SERVINGS
20 MINUTES
35 MINUTES

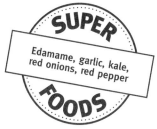

Edamame, garlic, kale,
red onions, red pepper

INGREDIENTS

8 cups (2 liters) vegetable broth

1 cup (250 ml) chopped **kale,** stems removed

1 leek, sliced

1 cup (250 ml) carrots, cut in small sticks

1½ cups (375 ml) whole mushrooms

1 **red pepper,** diced

1 small **red onion,** minced

3 green onions, minced

4 cloves **garlic,** minced

1 tbsp minced fresh ginger

1 cup (250 ml) shelled frozen **edamame**

1 tbsp miso

Seasoning to taste

METHOD

In a saucepan over medium heat, bring all ingredients to a boil except edamame, miso and seasonings. Cover and let simmer on medium heat, about 25 minutes.

Add edamame and continue cooking for 7 minutes.

Add miso and season to taste.

Nutrition Facts Per serving (⅙ of recipe)		
Amount		**% Daily Value**
Calories 280		
Fat 4 g		6%
Saturated 1 g + Trans 0 g		
Polyunsaturated 0.5 g		
Omega-6 0.5 g		
Omega-3 0.1 g		
Monounsaturated 3.1 g		
Cholesterol 0 mg		0%
Sodium 560 mg		23%
Potassium 1440 mg		41%
Carbohydrates 50 g		17%
Fiber 13 g		52%
Sugar 19 g		
Protein 12 g		
Vitamin A 2926 ER		290%
Vitamin C 77 mg		130%
Calcium 298 mg		25%
Iron 4.1 mg		30%
Phosphorus 201.2 mg		20%

REVITALIZING
MINESTRONE

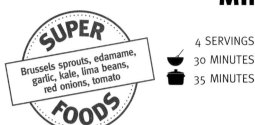

SUPER FOODS

Brussels sprouts, edamame, garlic, kale, lima beans, red onions, tomato

4 SERVINGS
30 MINUTES
35 MINUTES

INGREDIENTS

1 tbsp olive oil

1 small **red onion**, chopped

1 clove **garlic**, minced

1 carrot, chopped

1 stalk celery, chopped

1 can (28 oz/796 ml) Italian crushed **tomatoes**

2 cups (500 ml) beef broth

2 cups (500 ml) water

1 cup (250 ml) chopped **kale**, stems removed

1 cup (250 ml) **Brussels sprouts**, halved

¼ cup (60 ml) quinoa, rinsed and drained

1 can (19 oz/540 ml) **lima beans**, drained and rinsed

½ cup (125 ml) shelled frozen **edamame**

1 tsp dried sage

1 tsp dried thyme

1 tsp dried rosemary

¼ cup (60 ml) chopped fresh parsley

1 tbsp freshly grated Parmesan

Seasoning to taste

METHOD

In a large saucepan, heat oil over high heat and sauté onion, garlic, carrot and celery for a few minutes. Add tomatoes, broth, water, kale and Brussels sprouts. Continue cooking for about 20 minutes.

Add quinoa, lima beans, edamame, sage, thyme and rosemary. Continue cooking for about 12 minutes. Add water, if needed.

Before serving, add parsley and Parmesan. Season to taste.

Nutrition Facts Per serving	
Amount	**% Daily Value**
Calories 330	
Fat 7 g	11%
Saturated 1.5 g	
+ Trans 0 g	
Polyunsaturated 0.5 g	
Omega-6 0.5 g	
Omega-3 0.1 g	
Monounsaturated 0.4 g	
Cholesterol 1 mg	0%
Sodium 510 mg	21%
Potassium 1100 mg	32%
Carbohydrates 51 g	17%
Fiber 11 g	44%
Sugar 5 g	
Protein 16 g	
Vitamin A 1101 ER	110%
Vitamin C 65 mg	110%
Calcium 225 mg	20%
Iron 6.2 mg	45%
Phosphorus 248.5 mg	25%

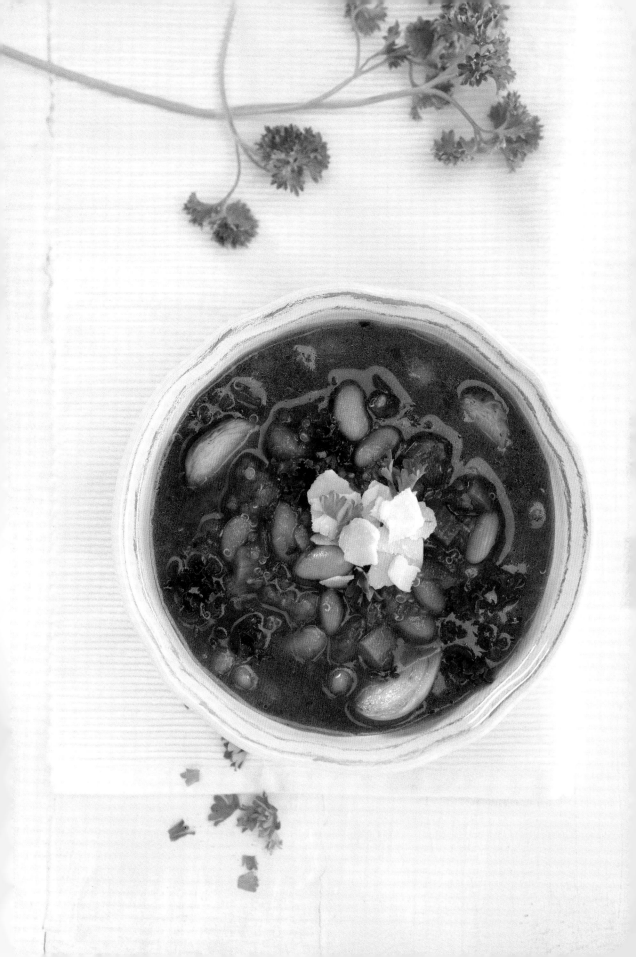

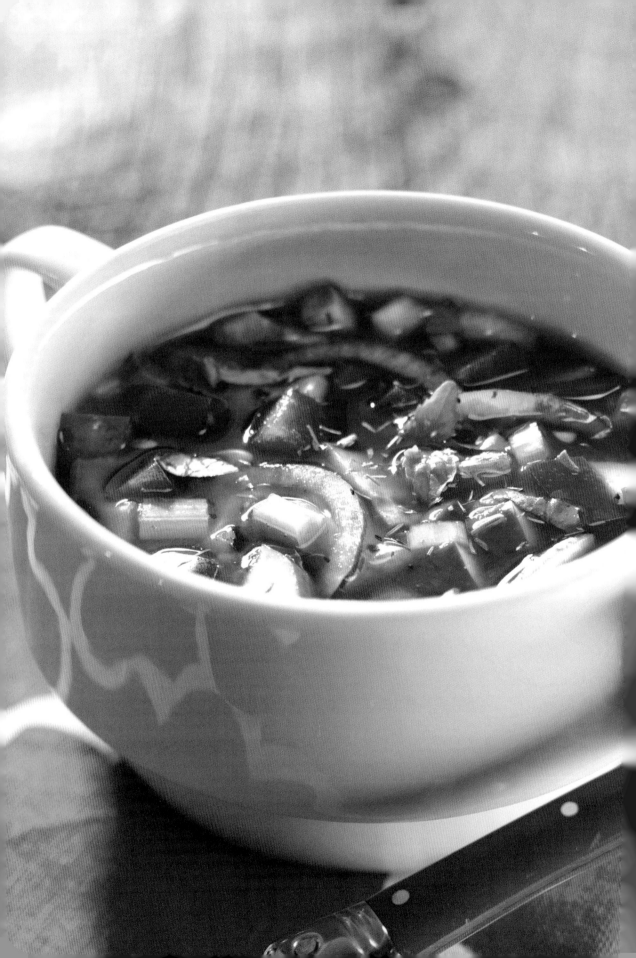

TOMATO
GAZPACHO

4 SERVINGS
15 MINUTES
2 HOURS

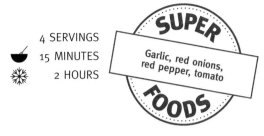

Garlic, red onions, red pepper, tomato

INGREDIENTS

2 cups (500 ml) **tomato** juice

1 **red pepper**, diced

1 cucumber, diced

1 stalk celery, diced

1 small **red onion**, minced

1 clove **garlic**, minced

2 tbsp chopped fresh basil

¼ tsp dried sage

1 tbsp olive oil

½ tsp Worcestershire sauce

2 drops Tabasco

Seasoning to taste

METHOD

In a bowl, combine all ingredients.

Refrigerate for at least 2 hours.

Serve cold.

TOMATOES: FRESH, COOKED, JUICED OR PASTE?

The amount of lycopene absorbed by the body is greater when consuming tomatoes in paste form as opposed to juice form. However, the highest absorption of lycopene occurs when you eat fresh tomatoes. When cooking with fresh tomatoes, it's always best to use a bit of olive oil. In fact, when heated, the lycopene found in tomatoes is more easily released, making it easier for the body to absorb, especially as it is fat-soluble. When consumed raw, your best bet is to cut tomatoes into small pieces and serve with a source of fat for better absorption of the lycopene.

Nutrition Facts Per serving	
Amount	**% Daily Value**
Calories 110	
Fat 3.5 g	5%
Saturated 0.5 g	
+ Trans 0 g	
Polyunsaturated 0.2 g	
Omega-6 0.1 g	
Omega-3 0 g	
Monounsaturated 0 g	
Cholesterol 0 mg	0%
Sodium 370 mg	15%
Potassium 580 mg	16%
Carbohydrates 16 g	5%
Fiber 3 g	12%
Sugar 9 g	
Protein 3 g	
Vitamin A 139 ER	15%
Vitamin C 53 mg	90%
Calcium 56 mg	6%
Iron 1.2 mg	8%
Phosphorus 70.7 mg	6%

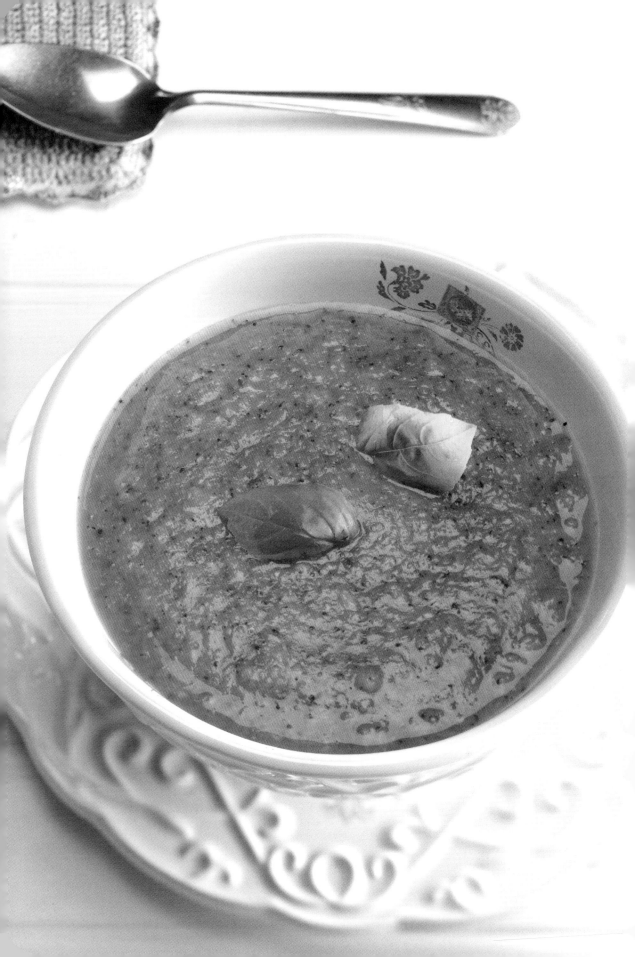

BROCCOLI
SOUP

4 TO 6 SERVINGS
15 MINUTES
30 MINUTES

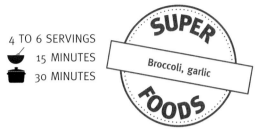

SUPER FOODS
Broccoli, garlic

INGREDIENTS

4 cups (1 liter) vegetable broth

3 cups (750 ml) **broccoli** florets

1 leek, sliced

1 stalk celery, chopped

1 sweet potato, diced

2 cloves **garlic**, minced

1 tsp fresh thyme

1 tsp coarsely chopped fresh basil

1 bay leaf

Seasoning to taste

Fresh basil, for garnish

METHOD

In a large saucepan over medium heat, combine all ingredients except seasonings and basil for garnish. Cook for about 30 minutes. Remove from heat, remove bay leaf and let cool.

In a blender (or directly in pot using an immersion blender), blend soup until smooth. Add water, if needed, and season to taste.

Garnish with basil before serving.

HOW TO SELECT BROCCOLI

The more vibrant green the broccoli, the more nutrient-rich it is. Avoid broccoli with yellowish heads, as yellowing is a sign it's lacking in beta-carotenes. Choose firm, strong stems, small compact florets and leaves that haven't flowered yet. A gap in the center of the head indicates the broccoli is past its prime.

Nutrition Facts Per serving (⅙ of recipe)	
Amount	% Daily Value
Calories 110	
Fat 0.5 g	1%
Saturated 0.1 g	
+ Trans 0 g	
Polyunsaturated 0.1 g	
Omega-6 0.1 g	
Omega-3 0.1 g	
Monounsaturated 0 g	
Cholesterol 0 mg	0%
Sodium 105 mg	4%
Potassium 450 mg	13%
Carbohydrates 23 g	8%
Fiber 5 g	20%
Sugar 5 g	
Protein 4 g	
Vitamin A 660 ER	70%
Vitamin C 72 mg	120%
Calcium 106 mg	10%
Iron 1.9 mg	15%
Phosphorus 88.5 mg	8%

CREAMY BUTTERNUT SQUASH
AND EDAMAME SOUP

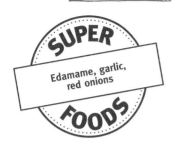

SUPER FOODS

Edamame, garlic, red onions

4 TO 6 SERVINGS

15 MINUTES

50 MINUTES

INGREDIENTS

1 butternut squash

1 tbsp olive oil

1 small **red onion**, minced

2 cloves **garlic**, minced

1 cup (250 ml) shelled frozen **edamame**

1 apple, peeled, cored and chopped

1 tsp minced fresh ginger

6 cups (1.5 liters) chicken or vegetable broth

Pinch ground nutmeg

1 bay leaf

Seasoning to taste

METHOD

Preheat oven to 350°F (180°C). Oil a baking sheet.

Cut squash in half lengthwise and remove seeds. Place squash facedown on prepared baking sheet. Cook in preheated oven for 30 minutes or until flesh is tender. Remove from oven and let cool. Scoop out flesh and set aside.

In a large saucepan, heat oil over medium heat and sauté onion and garlic for about 10 minutes or until onion becomes translucent. Add squash, edamame, apple, ginger, broth, nutmeg and bay leaf. Bring to a boil. Reduce heat to low. Let simmer for about 10 minutes. Remove bay leaf.

In a blender (or directly in pot using an immersion blender), blend soup until smooth. Add water, if needed, and season to taste.

Nutrition Facts Per serving (⅙ of recipe)	
Amount	**% Daily Value**
Calories 310	
Fat 6 g	9%
Saturated 1 g	
+ Trans 0 g	
Polyunsaturated 0.4 g	
Omega-6 0.3 g	
Omega-3 0 g	
Monounsaturated 0 g	
Cholesterol 0 mg	0%
Sodium 360 mg	15%
Potassium 1450 mg	42%
Carbohydrates 53 g	18%
Fiber 12 g	48%
Sugar 17 g	
Protein 10 g	
Vitamin A 4054 ER	410%
Vitamin C 64 mg	110%
Calcium 281 mg	25%
Iron 4.1 mg	30%
Phosphorus 167.5 mg	15%

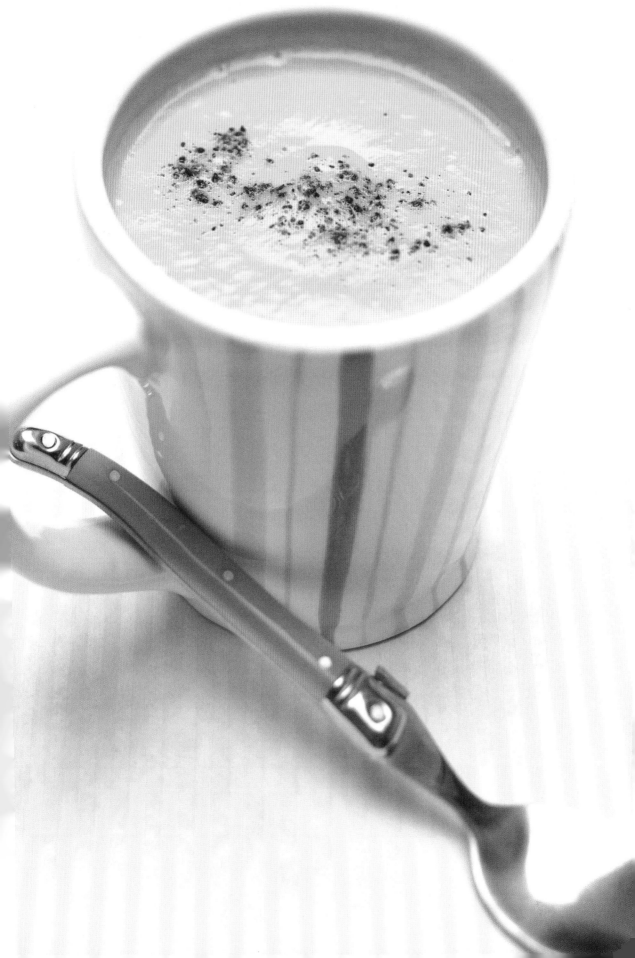

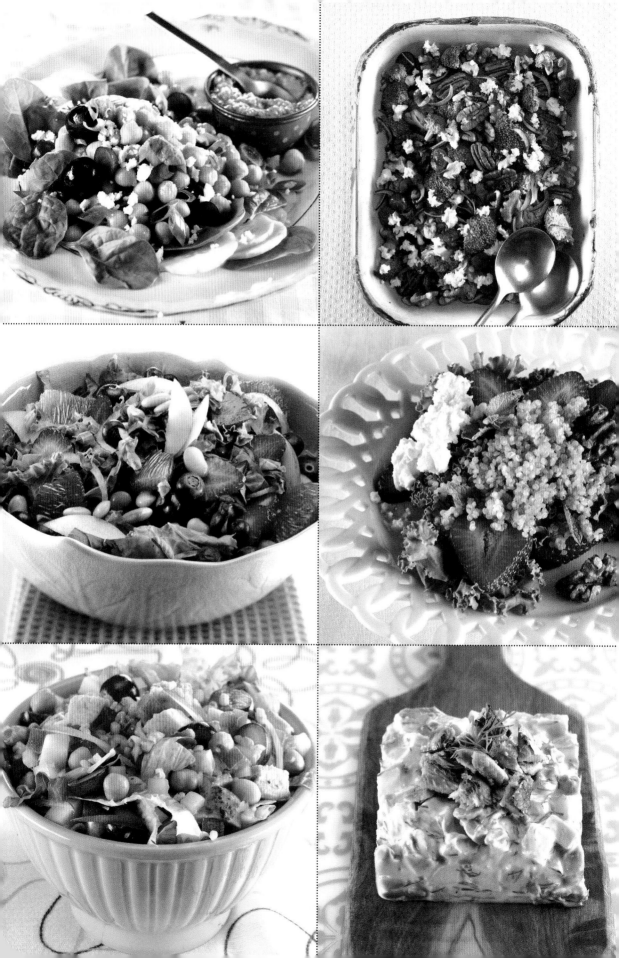

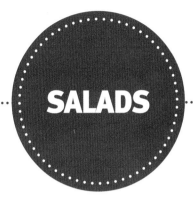

SALADS

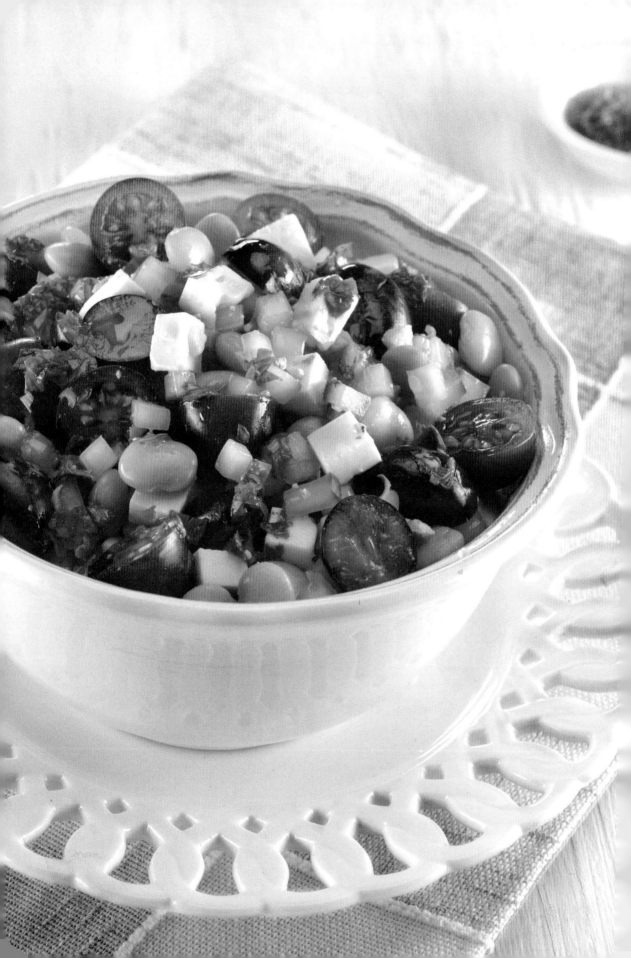

LIMA BEAN
GREEK SALAD

6 SERVINGS
15 MINUTES
30 MINUTES

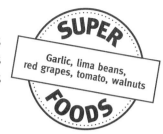

Garlic, lima beans, red grapes, tomato, walnuts

INGREDIENTS

20 cherry **tomatoes,** halved

½ cucumber, finely diced

1 can (19 oz/540 ml) **lima beans,** drained and rinsed

½ cup (125 ml) pitted black Kalamata olives

½ cup (125 ml) **red grapes,** halved

1 cup (250 ml) cubed feta cheese

¼ cup (60 ml) chopped **walnuts**

3 green onions, finely sliced

2 cloves **garlic,** minced

For the vinaigrette

3 tbsp olive oil

1 tbsp red wine vinegar

Juice of 1 lemon

¼ cup (60 ml) chopped fresh basil

1 tbsp chopped fresh cilantro

1 tbsp chopped fresh parsley

Seasoning to taste

METHOD

In a salad bowl, mix all ingredients for salad.

In a smaller bowl, whisk together ingredients for vinaigrette.

Pour vinaigrette on salad and toss to coat. Refrigerate for 30 minutes for extra flavor.

Nutrition Facts Per serving	
Amount	**% Daily Value**
Calories 290	
Fat 17 g	26%
Saturated 6 g	
+ Trans 0 g	
Polyunsaturated 3 g	
Omega-6 2 g	
Omega-3 0.5 g	
Monounsaturated 2.5 g	
Cholesterol 25 mg	8%
Sodium 430 mg	18%
Potassium 590 mg	17%
Carbohydrates 23 g	8%
Fiber 5 g	20%
Sugar 6 g	
Protein 10 g	
Vitamin A 131 ER	15%
Vitamin C 22 mg	35%
Calcium 205 mg	20%
Iron 2.8 mg	20%
Phosphorus 211.3 mg	20%

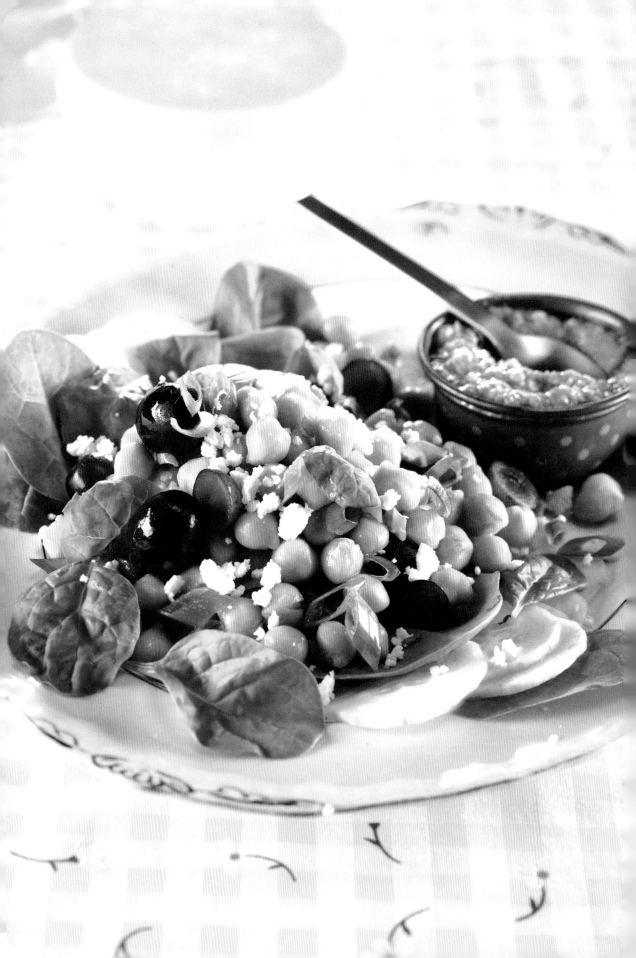

SPINACH AND
CHICKPEA SALAD

🥣 4 SERVINGS
15 MINUTES

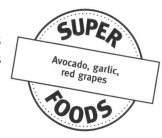

SUPER FOODS

Avocado, garlic, red grapes

INGREDIENTS

4 cups (1 liter) baby spinach

1 can (19 oz/540 ml) chickpeas, drained and rinsed

1 cup (250 ml) **red grapes**, halved

½ cup (125 ml) whole pitted black olives

½ cup (125 ml) crumbled light feta cheese

1 cucumber, peeled and sliced

3 green onions, thinly sliced

For the vinaigrette

2 tbsp olive oil

Juice of ½ lemon

1 ripe **avocado**, mashed

1 clove **garlic**, minced

Seasoning to taste

METHOD

In a salad bowl, mix all ingredients for salad.

In a smaller bowl, whisk together ingredients for vinaigrette.

Drizzle vinaigrette on salad before serving and toss to coat.

Nutrition Facts Per serving	
Amount	% Daily Value
Calories 450	
Fat 22 g	34%
Saturated 5 g	
+ Trans 0 g	
Polyunsaturated 2 g	
Omega-6 1.5 g	
Omega-3 0.2 g	
Monounsaturated 7 g	
Cholesterol 20 mg	7%
Sodium 820 mg	34%
Potassium 880 mg	25%
Carbohydrates 50 g	17%
Fiber 12 g	48%
Sugar 9 g	
Protein 13 g	
Vitamin A 348 ER	35%
Vitamin C 31 mg	50%
Calcium 230 mg	20%
Iron 4.3 mg	30%
Phosphorus 266.8 mg	25%

CHEF'S TIP

The best way to enjoy grapes is to remove them from the refrigerator at least 30 minutes prior to serving.

SPINACH AND ARUGULA SALAD
WITH SALMON

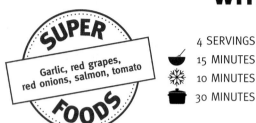

SUPER FOODS

Garlic, red grapes, red onions, salmon, tomato

4 SERVINGS

15 MINUTES

10 MINUTES

30 MINUTES

INGREDIENTS

1 sweet potato, cut in small cubes

2 cans (each 7.5 oz/213 g) **salmon,** drained and flaked

2 Italian **tomatoes,** chopped

1 cup (250 ml) **red grapes,** halved

1 small **red onion,** minced

1 clove **garlic,** minced

2 cups (500 ml) arugula

2 cups (500 ml) baby spinach

2 tbsp olive oil

Juice of ½ lemon

¼ cup (60 ml) coarsely chopped fresh basil

Seasoning to taste

METHOD

In a saucepan of boiling water over medium-low heat, cook sweet potato for 6 to 10 minutes. Drain and let cool in the refrigerator for at least 30 minutes.

Meanwhile, mix remaining ingredients in a salad bowl.

Add sweet potato and toss.

Nutrition Facts Per serving		
Amount		**% Daily Value**
Calories 250		
Fat 13 g		20%
Saturated 2.5 g		
+ Trans 0 g		
Polyunsaturated 2.5 g		
Omega-6 0.3 g		
Omega-3 1.5 g		
Monounsaturated 2.5 g		
Cholesterol 20 mg		7%
Sodium 420 mg		17%
Potassium 630 mg		18%
Carbohydrates 18 g		6%
Fiber 2 g		8%
Sugar 8 g		
Protein 15 g		
Vitamin A 645 ER		60%
Vitamin C 16 mg		25%
Calcium 226 mg		20%
Iron 1.9 mg		15%
Phosphorus 917.7 mg		80%

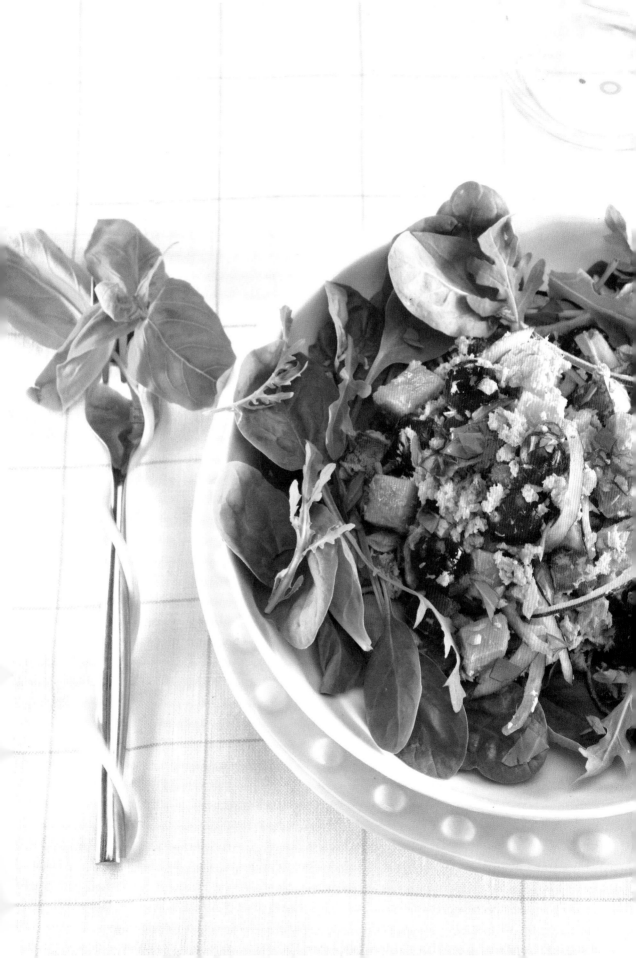

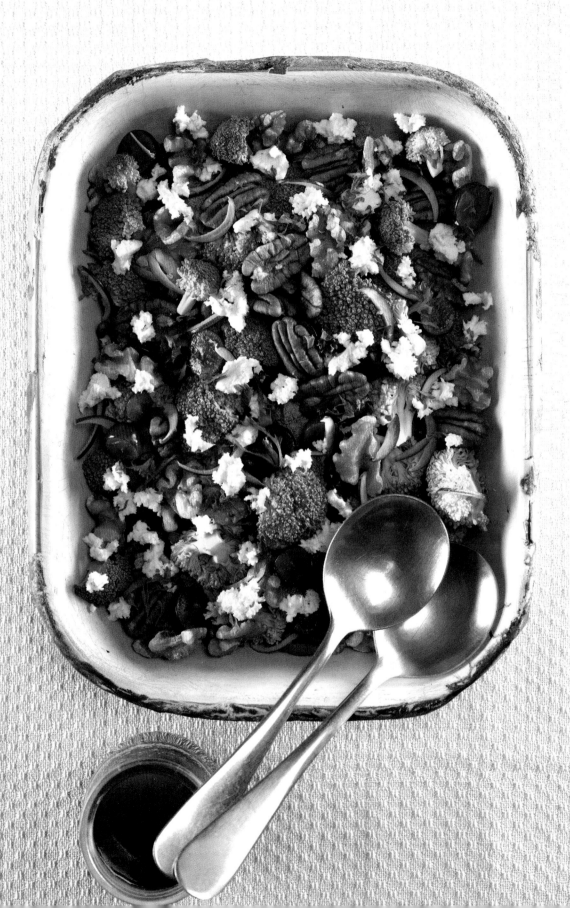

BROCCOLI SALAD WITH RED GRAPES
AND GOAT CHEESE

4 SERVINGS
20 MINUTES

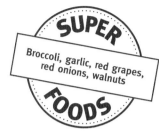

Broccoli, garlic, red grapes, red onions, walnuts

INGREDIENTS

2 cups (500 ml) **broccoli** florets

1 cup (250 ml) **red grapes**, halved

¾ cup (180 ml) crumbled goat cheese

½ cup (125 ml) **walnuts**

½ cup (125 ml) pecans

1 small **red onion**, minced

1 tbsp coarsely chopped fresh parsley

For the vinaigrette

4 tbsp balsamic vinegar

2 tbsp olive oil

2 tbsp maple syrup

2 tbsp Dijon mustard

2 tbsp lemon juice

1 clove **garlic**, minced

Seasoning to taste

METHOD

In a salad bowl, mix all ingredients for salad.

In a smaller bowl, whisk together ingredients for vinaigrette.

Drizzle vinaigrette on salad before serving and toss to coat.

Nutrition Facts Per serving		
Amount		**% Daily Value**
Calories 480		
Fat 35 g		54%
Saturated 10 g		
+ Trans 0 g		
Polyunsaturated 10 g		
Omega-6 8 g		
Omega-3 1.5 g		
Monounsaturated 13 g		
Cholesterol 30 mg		10%
Sodium 260 mg		11%
Potassium 410 mg		12%
Carbohydrates 26 g		9%
Fiber 4 g		16%
Sugar 18 g		
Protein 14 g		
Vitamin A 193 ER		20%
Vitamin C 51 mg		80%
Calcium 339 mg		30%
Iron 2.2 mg		15%
Phosphorus 339.8 mg		30%

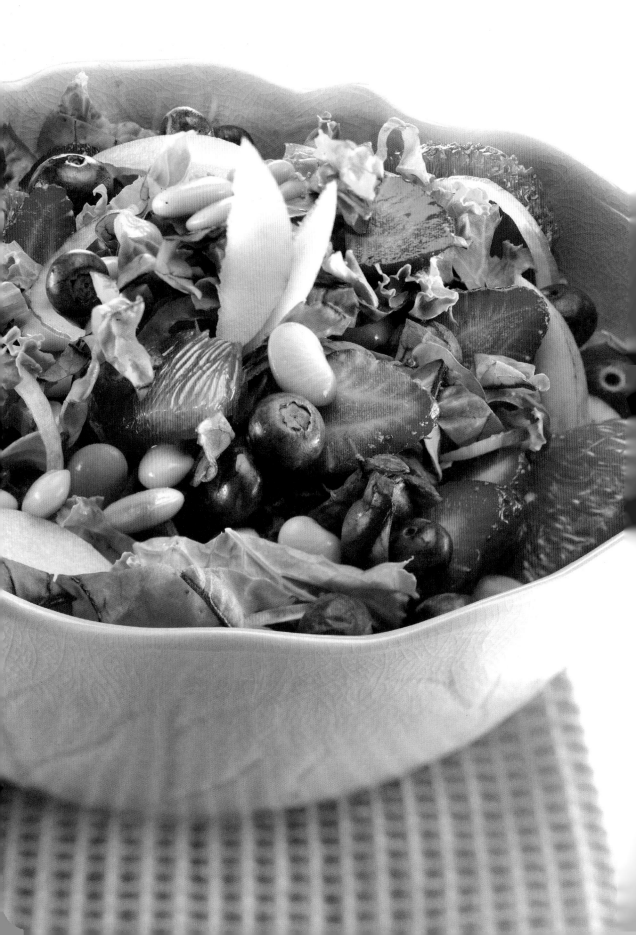

KALE, SWISS CHARD AND
LIMA BEAN SALAD

4 SERVINGS
20 MINUTES

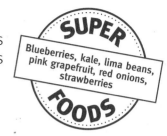

SUPER FOODS

Blueberries, kale, lima beans, pink grapefruit, red onions, strawberries

INGREDIENTS

1 can (19 oz/540 ml) **lima beans,** drained and rinsed

2 cups (500 ml) chopped **kale,** stems removed

2 cups (500 ml) chopped Swiss chard

1 small **red onion,** minced

1 pear, cored and sliced

½ **pink grapefruit,** cut in segments

1 cup (250 ml) sliced **strawberries**

1 cup (250 ml) **blueberries**

For the vinaigrette

1 tbsp maple syrup

1 tbsp olive oil

1 tsp balsamic vinegar

2 tsp Dijon mustard

Juice of 1 lemon

Seasoning to taste

METHOD

In a salad bowl, mix all ingredients for salad.

In a smaller bowl, whisk together ingredients for vinaigrette.

Drizzle vinaigrette on salad before serving and toss to coat.

DID YOU KNOW?

Legumes can help you lose weight. They make for a nourishing and satisfying meal, are high in fiber and low in fat.

Nutrition Facts Per serving	
Amount	**% Daily Value**
Calories 270	
Fat 8 g	12%
Saturated 0.5 g	
+ Trans 0 g	
Polyunsaturated 3.5 g	
Omega-6 1 g	
Omega-3 0.2 g	
Monounsaturated 3.5 g	
Cholesterol 0 mg	0%
Sodium 230 mg	9%
Potassium 7580 mg	217%
Carbohydrates 520 g	173%
Fiber 75 g	300%
Sugar 218 g	
Protein 51 g	
Vitamin A 439 ER	45%
Vitamin C 370 mg	620%
Calcium 1156 mg	110%
Iron 11.9 mg	80%
Phosphorus 1409.3 mg	130%

QUINOA SALAD WITH KALE
AND STRAWBERRIES

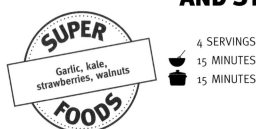

SUPER FOODS

Garlic, kale, strawberries, walnuts

4 SERVINGS

15 MINUTES

15 MINUTES

INGREDIENTS

½ cup (125 ml) water

¼ cup (60 ml) quinoa, rinsed and drained

2 cups (500 ml) chopped **kale**, stems removed

1 cup (250 ml) **strawberries**, quartered

¼ cup (60 ml) **walnuts**, roasted

¼ cup (60 ml) goat cheese, in pieces

3 tbsp chopped fresh mint

For the vinaigrette

3 tbsp balsamic vinegar

2 tbsp olive oil

2 tbsp maple syrup

1 clove **garlic**, minced

Seasoning to taste

METHOD

In a large saucepan over medium heat, bring water to a boil and add quinoa. Reduce heat to low. Cover and let simmer for 12 minutes. Drain and let cool.

In a salad bowl, mix all ingredients for salad.

In a smaller bowl, whisk together ingredients for vinaigrette.

Drizzle vinaigrette on salad before serving and toss to coat.

Nutrition Facts Per serving	
Amount	**% Daily Value**
Calories 260	
Fat 15 g	23%
Saturated 4 g	
+ Trans 0 g	
Polyunsaturated 4 g	
Omega-6 3.5 g	
Omega-3 0.5 g	
Monounsaturated 6 g	
Cholesterol 10 mg	3%
Sodium 50 mg	2%
Potassium 290 mg	8%
Carbohydrates 25 g	8%
Fiber 4 g	16%
Sugar 10 g	
Protein 7 g	
Vitamin A 298 ER	30%
Vitamin C 40 mg	70%
Calcium 184 mg	15%
Iron 2.1 mg	15%
Phosphorus 164.9 mg	15%

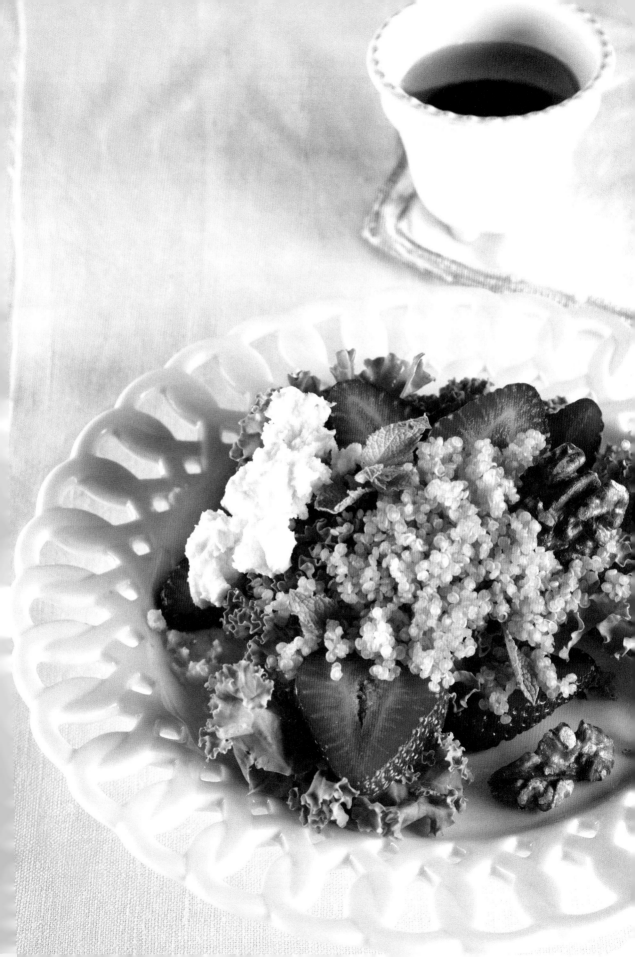

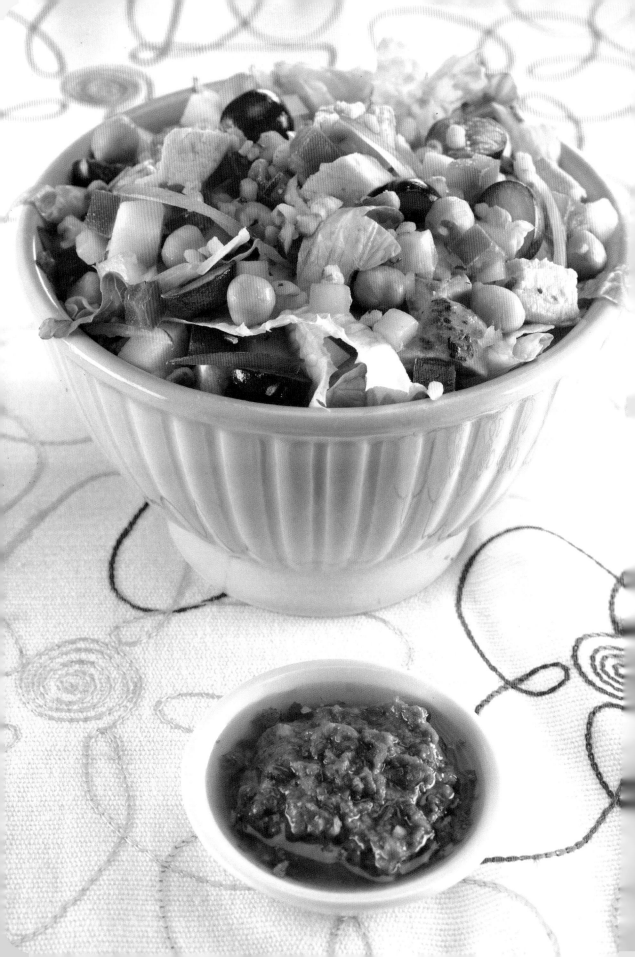

CHICKEN SALAD WITH
AVOCADO AND WALNUTS

6 SERVINGS

20 MINUTES

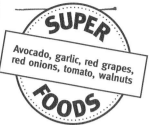

SUPER FOODS

Avocado, garlic, red grapes, red onions, tomato, walnuts

INGREDIENTS

4 cups (1 liter) chopped lettuce

1 lb (454 g) cooked chicken breast, chopped

1 can (19 oz/540 ml) chickpeas, drained and rinsed

1 apple, peeled, cored and chopped

1 cucumber, peeled and chopped

1 **tomato**, chopped

1 stalk celery, finely chopped

1 small **red onion**, minced

½ cup (125 ml) **red grapes**, halved

2 tbsp coarsely chopped **walnuts**

For the vinaigrette

3 tbsp olive oil

Juice of 1 lemon

1 ripe **avocado**, mashed

1 clove **garlic**, minced

2 tbsp coarsely chopped fresh tarragon

Seasoning to taste

METHOD

In a salad bowl, mix all ingredients for salad.

In a smaller bowl, whisk together ingredients for vinaigrette.

Drizzle vinaigrette on salad before serving and toss to coat.

COMMON MISCONCEPTIONS

Avocados make you fat.

FALSE. Avocados are considered to be the fruit with the most calories, but they're filled with monounsaturated fat, otherwise known as the "good" fat. And avocados also contain fiber, which helps you feel fuller longer.

Nutrition Facts Per serving	
Amount	% Daily Value
Calories 420	
Fat 20 g	31%
Saturated 3.5 g	
+ Trans 0 g	
Polyunsaturated 4 g	
Omega-6 3.5 g	
Omega-3 0.4 g	
Monounsaturated 11 g	
Cholesterol 55 mg	18%
Sodium 80 mg	3%
Potassium 900 mg	26%
Carbohydrates 34 g	11%
Fiber 8 g	32%
Sugar 11 g	
Protein 27 g	
Vitamin A 280 ER	30%
Vitamin C 25 mg	40%
Calcium 95 mg	8%
Iron 4 mg	30%
Phosphorus 325.2 mg	30%

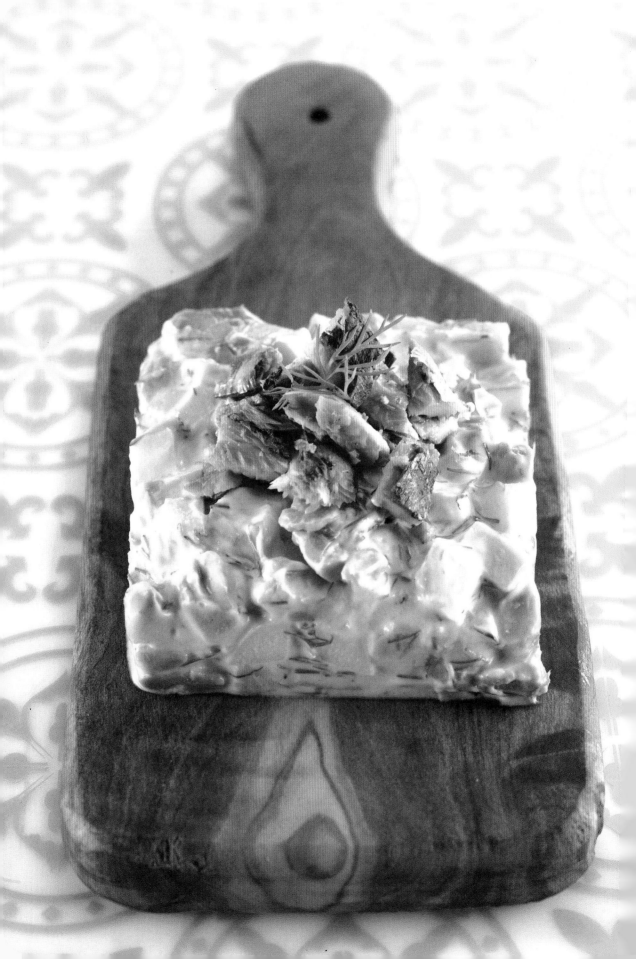

NORDIC SARDINE
SALAD

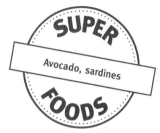

4 SERVINGS
10 MINUTES

Avocado, sardines

INGREDIENTS

1 green apple, chopped

1 **avocado**, chopped

½ cup (125 ml) plain yogurt

1 tbsp chopped dill

2 tbsp cider vinegar
or lemon juice

Seasoning to taste

2 cans (each 3.5 oz/100 g)
sardines, chopped

METHOD

In a salad bowl, mix together apple, avocado, yogurt and dill.

Add vinegar and season to taste.

Serve topped with sardines.

Nutrition Facts Per serving	
Amount	**% Daily Value**
Calories 220	
Fat 13 g	20%
Saturated 2 g + Trans 0 g	
Polyunsaturated 3.5 g	
Omega-6 2.5 g	
Omega-3 1 g	
Monounsaturated 7 g	
Cholesterol 65 mg	22%
Sodium 260 mg	11%
Potassium 550 mg	16%
Carbohydrates 12 g	4%
Fiber 4 g	16%
Sugar 7 g	
Protein 14 g	
Vitamin A 30 ER	2%
Vitamin C 7 mg	10%
Calcium 244 mg	20%
Iron 1.7 mg	10%
Phosphorus 302.9 mg	30%

SAUTÉED VEGETABLE SALAD
WITH SARDINES

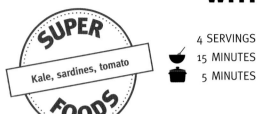

4 SERVINGS

15 MINUTES

5 MINUTES

INGREDIENTS

2 tbsp sesame or olive oil

2 green onions, finely chopped

2 **tomatoes**, diced

1 cup (250 ml) **kale**, stems removed, cut in strips

1 cup (250 ml) cucumber, peeled and cut in sticks

2 cans (each 3.5 oz/100 g) **sardines**, chopped

1 tbsp sesame seeds, for garnish

For the vinaigrette

⅓ cup (80 ml) olive oil

3 tbsp balsamic vinegar

3 tbsp low-sodium soy sauce

1 tbsp lemon juice

Seasoning to taste

METHOD

In a skillet, heat oil over medium-high heat and sauté onions, tomatoes, kale, cucumber and sardines for about 5 minutes. Place in salad bowl and set aside.

In a smaller bowl, whisk together ingredients for vinaigrette. Drizzle on sardine mixture.

Before serving, sprinkle salad with sesame seeds.

Nutrition Facts Per serving	
Amount	**% Daily Value**
Calories 370	
Fat 30 g	46%
Saturated 4 g	
+ Trans 0 g	
Polyunsaturated 5 g	
Omega-6 4.5 g	
Omega-3 1 g	
Monounsaturated 20 g	
Cholesterol 65 mg	22%
Sodium 650 mg	27%
Potassium 540 mg	15%
Carbohydrates 11 g	4%
Fiber 3 g	12%
Sugar 5 g	
Protein 14 g	
Vitamin A 203 ER	20%
Vitamin C 20 mg	35%
Calcium 237 mg	20%
Iron 2.6 mg	20%
Phosphorus 293.8 mg	25%

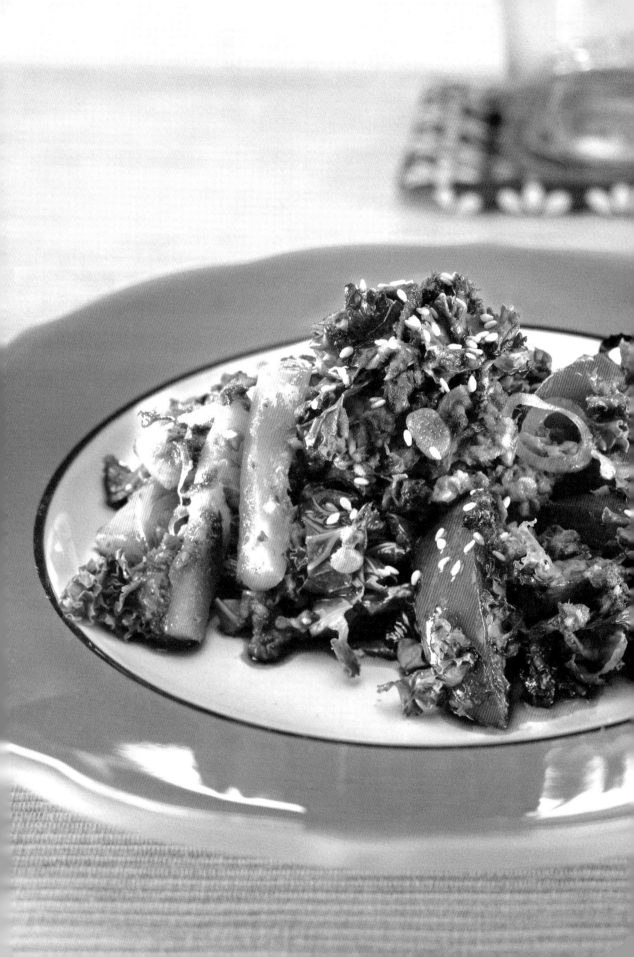

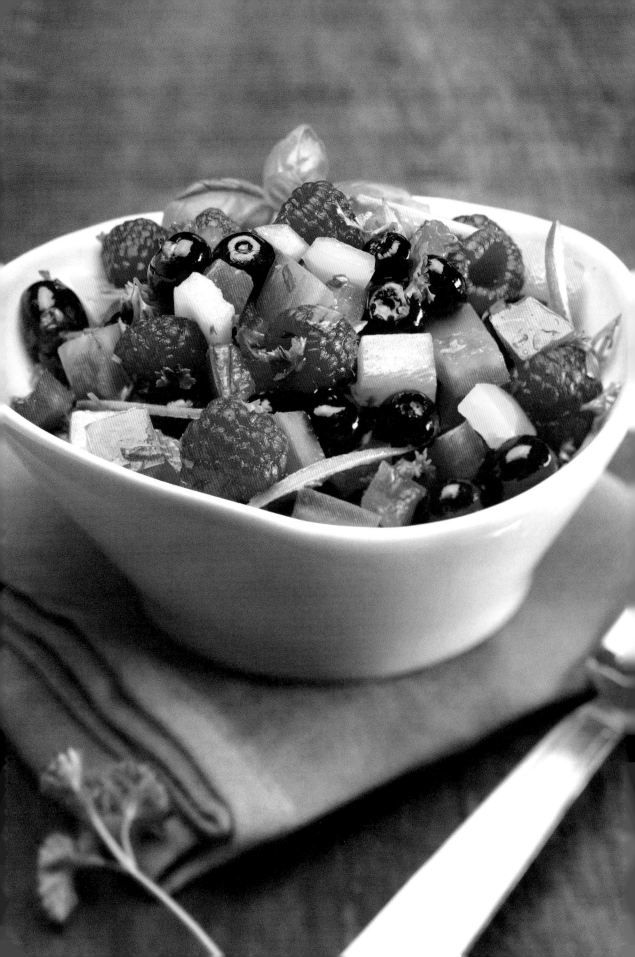

ANTIOXIDANT
SALAD

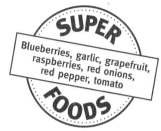

🥣 4 SERVINGS
15 MINUTES

SUPER FOODS

Blueberries, garlic, grapefruit, raspberries, red onions, red pepper, tomato

INGREDIENTS

1 **red pepper**, chopped

1 yellow pepper, chopped

6 Italian **tomatoes**, chopped

1 cup (250 ml) fresh **raspberries**

1 cup (250 ml) fresh **blueberries**

For the vinaigrette

2 tbsp olive oil

1 tbsp lemon juice

1 tbsp **grapefruit** juice (optional)

1 small **red onion**, minced

1 clove **garlic**, minced

¼ cup (60 ml) chopped fresh basil

1 tsp chopped fresh ginger

1 tbsp chopped fresh parsley

Seasoning to taste

METHOD

In a salad bowl, mix all ingredients for salad.

In a smaller bowl, whisk together ingredients for vinaigrette.

Drizzle vinaigrette on salad before serving and toss to coat.

Nutrition Facts Per serving	
Amount	**% Daily Value**
Calories 160	
Fat 7 g	11%
Saturated 1 g + Trans 0 g	
Polyunsaturated 0.4 g	
Omega-6 0.2 g	
Omega-3 0.1 g	
Monounsaturated 0.1 g	
Cholesterol 0 mg	0%
Sodium 10 mg	0%
Potassium 480 mg	14%
Carbohydrates 22 g	7%
Fiber 5 g	20%
Sugar 11 g	
Protein 3 g	
Vitamin A 164 ER	15%
Vitamin C 102 mg	170%
Calcium 48 mg	4%
Iron 1.1 mg	8%
Phosphorus 68.1 mg	6%

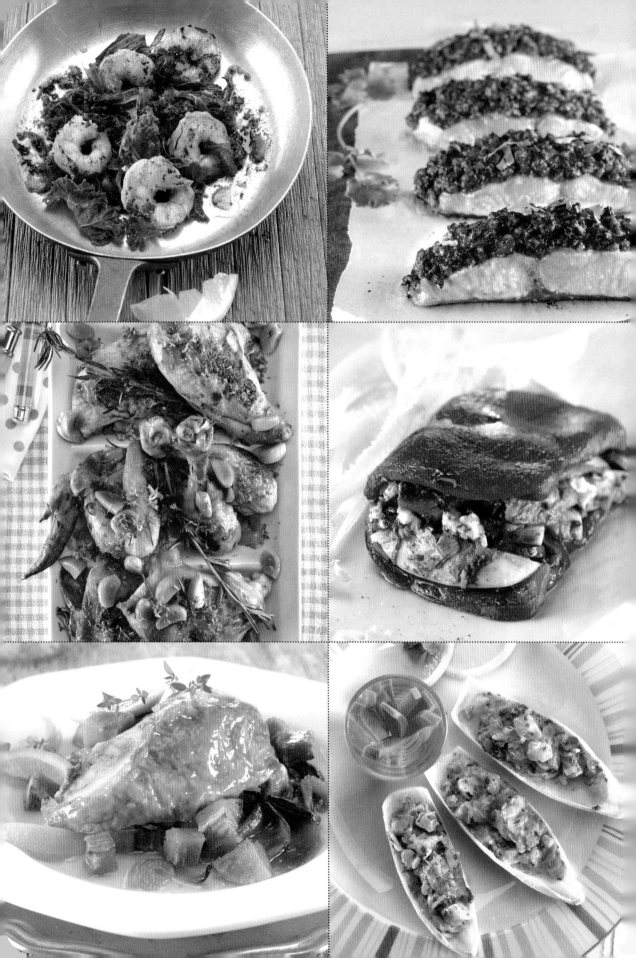

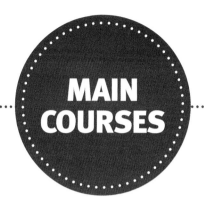

MAIN COURSES

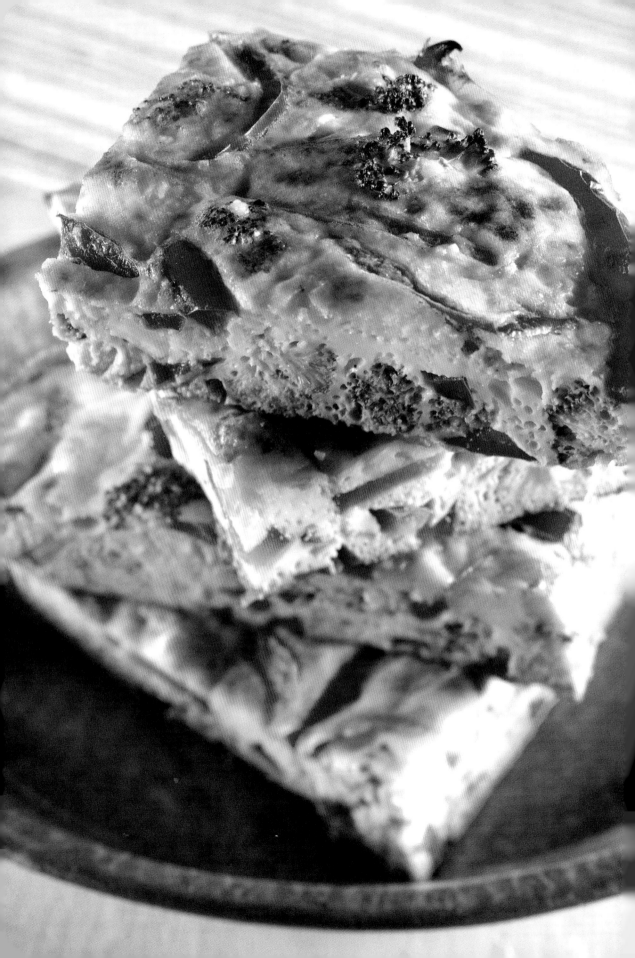

BROCCOLI
FRITTATA

4 SERVINGS
15 MINUTES
20 MINUTES

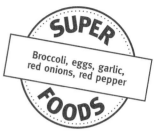

Broccoli, eggs, garlic, red onions, red pepper

INGREDIENTS

1 tbsp olive oil

1 small **red onion**, minced

2 cloves **garlic**, minced

2 **red peppers**, thinly sliced

1½ cups (375 ml) **broccoli** florets

8 **eggs**

½ cup (125 ml) milk

½ cup (125 ml) crumbled feta

METHOD

Preheat oven to 350°F (180°C).

In an ovenproof skillet, heat oil over medium heat and sauté onions, garlic, peppers and broccoli for about 5 minutes.

Meanwhile, in a bowl, whisk eggs. Add milk and cheese. Pour into skillet and stir for 2 minutes.

Continue cooking in preheated oven for 10 minutes or until eggs have set and frittata has risen.

Using a spatula, slide frittata onto a cutting board. Divide into 4 equal servings.

Nutrition Facts Per serving	
Amount	**% Daily Value**
Calories 310	
Fat 19 g	29%
Saturated 7 g	
+ Trans 0.1 g	
Polyunsaturated 2 g	
Omega-6 1.5 g	
Omega-3 0.2 g	
Monounsaturated 5 g	
Cholesterol 390 mg	132%
Sodium 370 mg	16%
Potassium 470 mg	13%
Carbohydrates 15 g	5%
Fiber 2 g	8%
Sugar 7 g	
Protein 19 g	
Vitamin A 320 ER	30%
Vitamin C 53 mg	90%
Calcium 235 mg	20%
Iron 1.9 mg	15%
Phosphorus 291.4 mg	25%

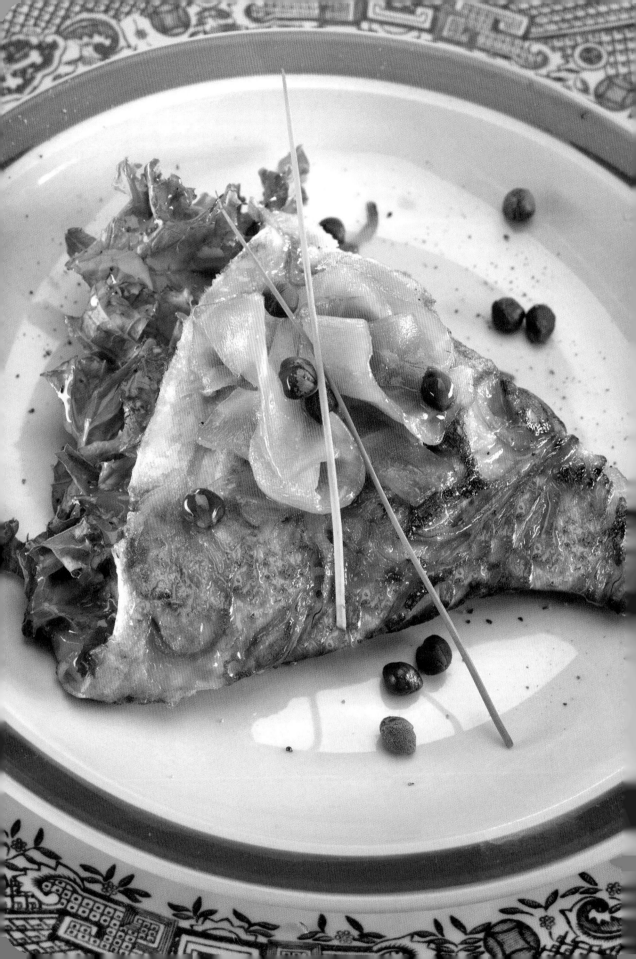

SMOKED SALMON
AND KALE OMELET

4 SERVINGS
15 MINUTES
10 MINUTES

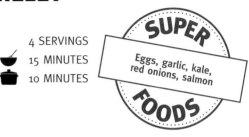

SUPER
FOODS

Eggs, garlic, kale,
red onions, salmon

INGREDIENTS

1 tbsp olive oil

1 small **red onion**, minced

1 clove **garlic**, minced

4 **eggs**, whisked

1 tbsp minced fresh chives

1 cup (250 ml) coarsely chopped
kale, stems removed

2 oz (60 g) smoked **salmon**,
thinly sliced

1 tbsp capers (optional)

METHOD

In a skillet, heat oil over medium-low heat and sauté onion and garlic for about 3 minutes.

Add eggs and chives. Stir and continue cooking for about 3 minutes.

Lay kale over omelet and fold omelet in half. Continue cooking for 1 minute.

Top with smoked salmon and capers, if using.

COMMON MISCONCEPTIONS
Eating eggs increases cholesterol.
FALSE. Old habits die hard. But scientific research has proven that dietary cholesterol, like the kind found in eggs, has very little influence on blood cholesterol.

Nutrition Facts Per serving	
Amount	% Daily Value
Calories 150	
Fat 9 g	14%
Saturated 2 g	
+ Trans 0 g	
Polyunsaturated 1 g	
Omega-6 1 g	
Omega-3 0.1 g	
Monounsaturated 2.5 g	
Cholesterol 190 mg	63%
Sodium 300 mg	12%
Potassium 200 mg	6%
Carbohydrates 7 g	2%
Fiber 1 g	4%
Sugar 2 g	
Protein 10 g	
Vitamin A 194 ER	20%
Vitamin C 11 mg	20%
Calcium 73 mg	6%
Iron 1 mg	6%
Phosphorus 113.2 mg	10%

SEARED SCALLOPS AND SHRIMP
WITH GRAPEFRUIT

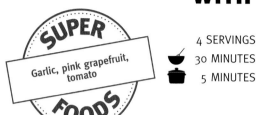

SUPER FOODS

Garlic, pink grapefruit, tomato

4 SERVINGS

30 MINUTES

5 MINUTES

INGREDIENTS

2 tbsp olive oil

4 green onions, finely chopped

1 clove **garlic**, minced

1 tbsp grated fresh ginger

12 oz (340 g) raw, medium shrimp, deveined

12 oz (340 g) scallops, trimmed (muscles removed)

½ **pink grapefruit**, cut in segments

2 oranges, cut in segments

1 lime, cut in segments

½ lemon, cut in segments

Drizzle maple syrup

12 cherry **tomatoes**, halved

Seasoning to taste

¼ cup (60 ml) chopped fresh cilantro

METHOD

In a large skillet, heat oil over high heat and sauté onions, garlic and ginger. Reduce heat to medium and add shrimp and scallops. Cook for 2 minutes on each side or until shrimp are pink and scallops are opaque.

Remove from heat. Add grapefruit, oranges, lime, lemon, maple syrup and tomatoes. Toss, season and garnish with cilantro.

Nutrition Facts Per serving	
Amount	**% Daily Value**
Calories 350	
Fat 9 g	14%
Saturated 1.5 g	
+ Trans 0 g	
Polyunsaturated 1 g	
Omega-6 0.2 g	
Omega-3 0.5 g	
Monounsaturated 0.4 g	
Cholesterol 190 mg	65%
Sodium 350 mg	14%
Potassium 1110 mg	32%
Carbohydrates 30 g	10%
Fiber 5 g	20%
Sugar 16 g	
Protein 36 g	
Vitamin A 210 ER	20%
Vitamin C 111 mg	190%
Calcium 203 mg	20%
Iron 6 mg	45%
Phosphorus 378.9 mg	35%

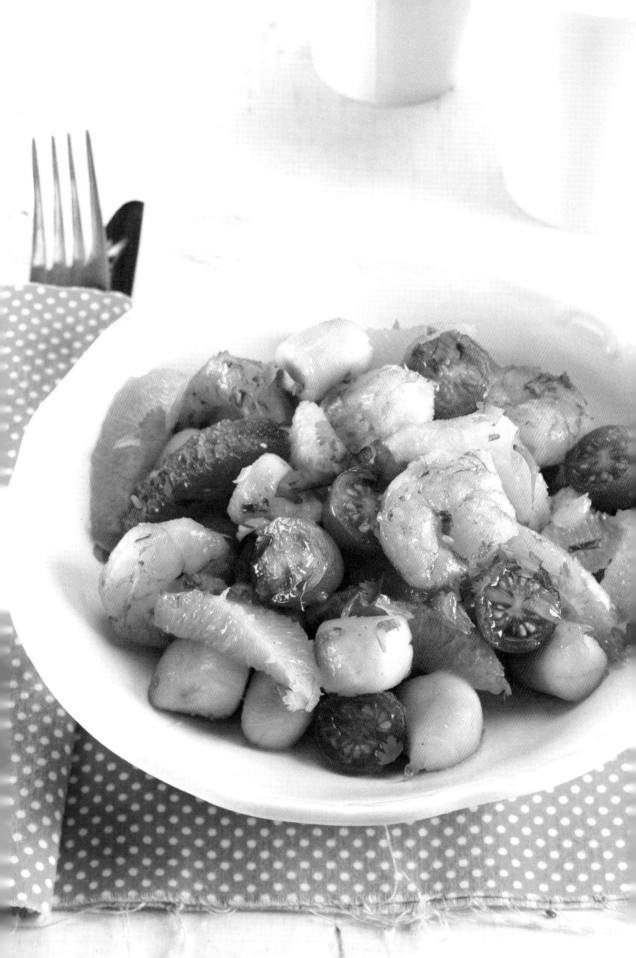

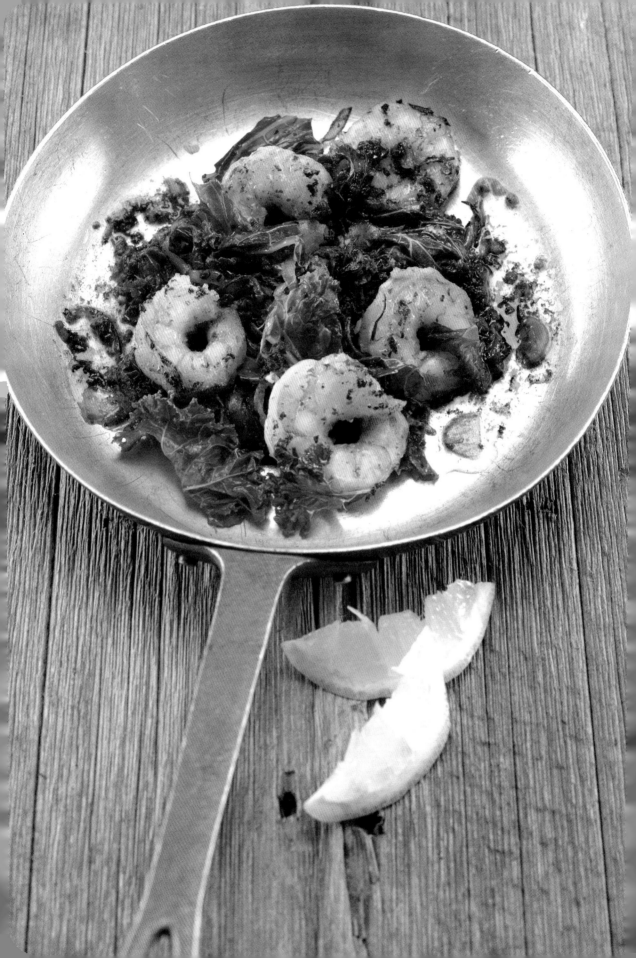

GINGER SHRIMP WITH
SAUTÉED KALE

4 SERVINGS
15 MINUTES
20 MINUTES
20 MINUTES

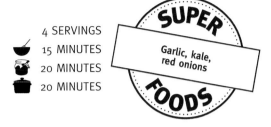

SUPER
Garlic, kale,
red onions
FOODS

INGREDIENTS

20 large shrimp (21–25 count), deveined

1 bunch **kale**, ribs removed, coarsely chopped

2 tbsp olive oil

1 small **red onion**, minced

1 clove **garlic**, minced

1 tbsp white wine

Seasoning to taste

1 tbsp lemon juice

For the marinade

Juice of 2 lemons

1 tsp olive oil

3 cloves **garlic**, minced

1 small **red onion**, minced

1 tbsp minced fresh ginger

1 tbsp chopped fresh cilantro

Seasoning to taste

METHOD

In a bowl, whisk together ingredients for marinade. Add shrimp and let sit for 20 minutes.

Meanwhile, cook kale in a saucepan of boiling water for 8 minutes or until kale is tender. Strain water and place kale on paper towel.

In a skillet, heat oil over high heat and sauté onion and garlic for 3 minutes. Reduce heat to medium and add kale and white wine. Season to taste and cook for another 2 minutes, adding water as needed.

In another skillet over high heat, sauté marinated shrimp for 1 minute. Reduce heat to medium and continue cooking, stirring constantly, for another 5 minutes.

Drizzle lemon juice on kale. Serve with ginger shrimp.

Nutrition Facts Per serving	
Amount	% Daily Value
Calories 210	
Fat 11 g	17%
Saturated 1.5 g	
+ Trans 0 g	
Polyunsaturated 0.3 g	
Omega-6 0.1 g	
Omega-3 0.1 g	
Monounsaturated 0.1 g	
Cholesterol 55 mg	18%
Sodium 75 mg	3%
Potassium 350 mg	10%
Carbohydrates 19 g	6%
Fiber 3 g	12%
Sugar 4 g	
Protein 9 g	
Vitamin A 255 ER	25%
Vitamin C 31 mg	50%
Calcium 128 mg	10%
Iron 1.7 mg	10%
Phosphorus 101.8 mg	10%

— DID YOU KNOW? —

To avoid watery eyes, peel onions under water, as the molecule responsible for your tears (syn-propanethial-S-oxide) is extremely soluble in water.

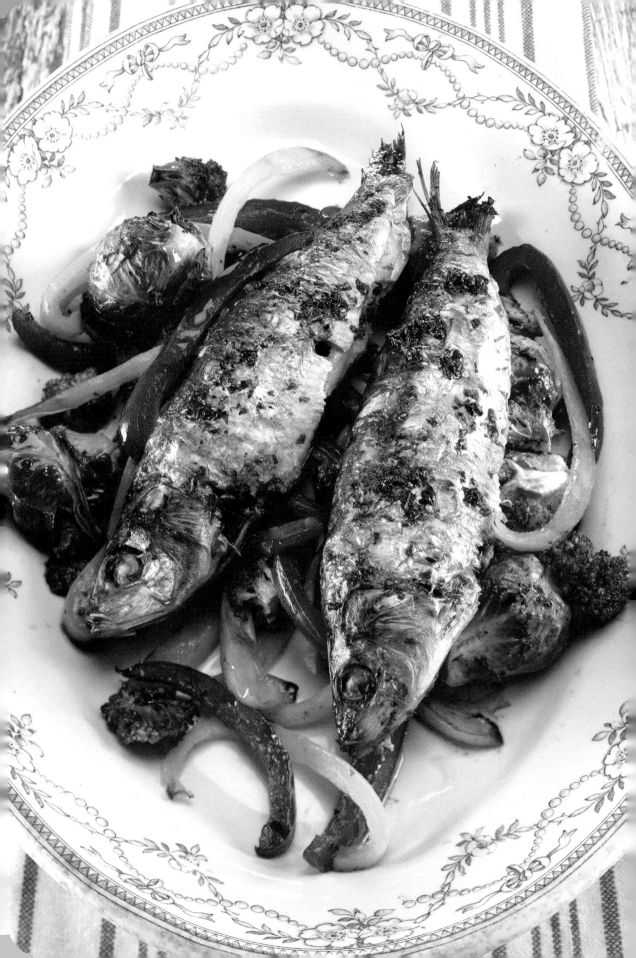

GRILLED VEGGIES AND SARDINES
À LA PORTUGUESE

4 SERVINGS
20 MINUTES
20 MINUTES

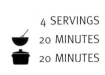

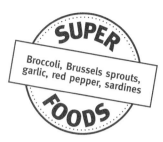

Broccoli, Brussels sprouts, garlic, red pepper, sardines

INGREDIENTS

1 package (28 oz/800 g) **sardines**, thawed

Pinch coarse salt

For the grilled vegetables

1 head **broccoli**, in florets

3 cups (750 ml) **Brussels sprouts**

2 cloves **garlic**, minced

1 **red pepper**, chopped

1 yellow pepper, chopped

2 tbsp olive oil

1 tbsp balsamic vinegar

2 tbsp lemon juice

½ tsp dried oregano

½ tsp dried basil

Leaves of 1 sprig fresh rosemary

Leaves of 1 sprig fresh thyme

Seasoning to taste

For the sauce

2 tbsp olive oil

1 tbsp lemon juice

4 cloves **garlic**, minced

¼ cup (60 ml) finely chopped fresh parsley

Pinch coarse sea salt

METHOD

Position rack in center of oven and preheat to 350°F (180°C).

Under cold running water, remove scales from sardines. Starting at tail and using the back of a knife, gently scrape skin toward head. Using scissors, cut off dorsal fins. Starting at the point where the tail meets the body, cut belly open and scrape out entrails. Place sardines on plate and sprinkle with coarse salt.

In a large bowl, mix all ingredients for the grilled vegetables. Place on a baking sheet and cook in center of preheated oven or barbecue for 20 minutes.

After 10 minutes, add sardines to baking sheet. Turn sardines partway through.

In a bowl, whisk together ingredients for sauce.

Serve grilled vegetables and sardines with sauce.

Nutrition Facts Per serving	
Amount	% Daily Value
Calories 240	
Fat 14 g	22%
Saturated 2 g	
+ Trans 0 g	
Polyunsaturated 0.3 g	
Omega-6 0.1 g	
Omega-3 0.1 g	
Monounsaturated 0 g	
Cholesterol 0 mg	0%
Sodium 30 mg	1%
Potassium 560 mg	16%
Carbohydrates 23 g	8%
Fiber 5 g	20%
Sugar 4 g	
Protein 5 g	
Vitamin A 159 ER	15%
Vitamin C 51 mg	80%
Calcium 117 mg	10%
Iron 2.4 mg	15%
Phosphorus 120.9 mg	10%

SARDINE-STUFFED
PEPPERS

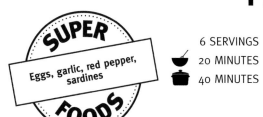

6 SERVINGS

20 MINUTES

40 MINUTES

INGREDIENTS

6 large **red peppers**, halved lengthwise, seeds removed

3 cans (each 3.5 oz/100 g) **sardines** packed in oil, drained

4 hard-boiled **eggs**, peeled and chopped in eight pieces

½ cup (125 ml) crumbled goat cheese

12 large pitted black olives, sliced

1 handful green salad

For the vinaigrette

2 tbsp olive oil

1 tbsp balsamic vinegar

1 clove **garlic**, minced

1 tsp grainy mustard

2 tbsp chopped fresh cilantro

Seasoning to taste

METHOD

Preheat oven to 400°F (200°C).

Place peppers on a baking sheet and bake in pre-heated oven for 40 minutes or until skin begins to wrinkle. Remove from oven and let cool before peeling.

Meanwhile, in a bowl, whisk together ingredients for vinaigrette. Add sardines, eggs, cheese and olives. Gently toss.

Divide mixture among peppers. Place one pepper half over the other to make a sandwich.

Serve with salad.

Nutrition Facts Per serving	
Amount	**% Daily Value**
Calories 300	
Fat 20 g	31%
Saturated 6 g	
+ Trans 0 g	
Polyunsaturated 3.5 g	
Omega-6 2.5 g	
Omega-3 1 g	
Monounsaturated 6 g	
Cholesterol 200 mg	68%
Sodium 600 mg	25%
Potassium 430 mg	12%
Carbohydrates 9 g	3%
Fiber 2 g	8%
Sugar 4 g	
Protein 21 g	
Vitamin A 373 ER	35%
Vitamin C 62 mg	100%
Calcium 361 mg	35%
Iron 3.6 mg	25%
Phosphorus 397 mg	35%

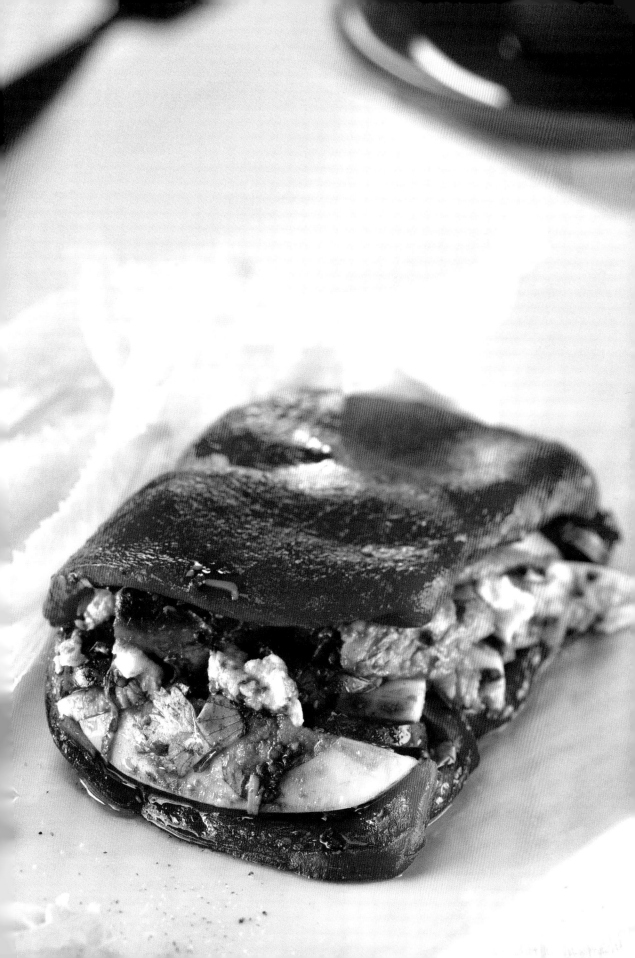

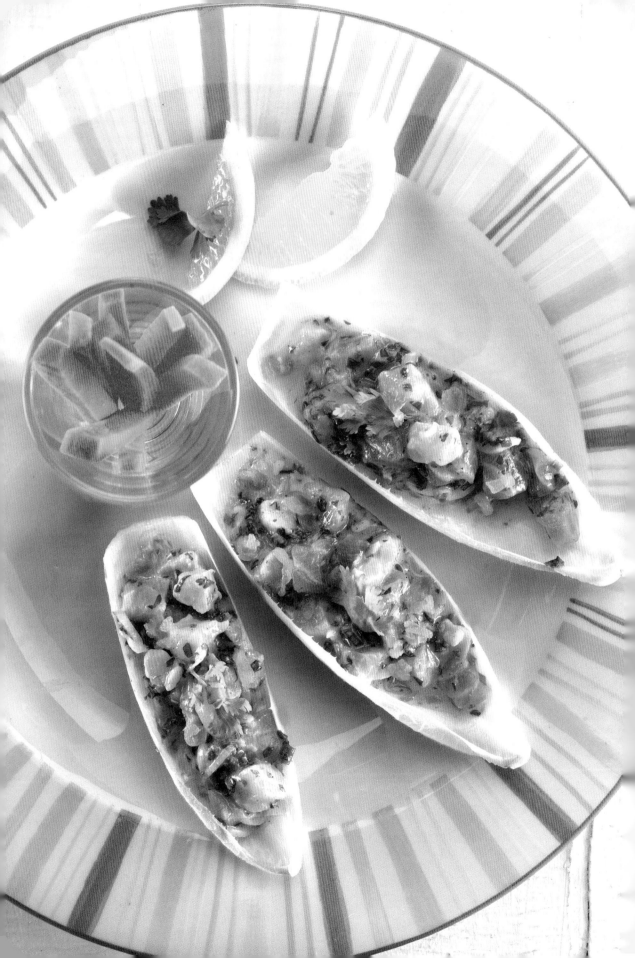

SALMON
TARTARE

6 SERVINGS
20 MINUTES

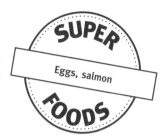

INGREDIENTS

1 lb 5 oz (600 g) skinless **salmon** filet, cubed

5 oz (150 g) smoked **salmon**, chopped

2 fresh **egg** yolks

2 tbsp Dijon mustard

1 tbsp maple syrup

2 tbsp freshly squeezed lemon juice

2 green onions, finely sliced

2 tbsp chopped fresh chives

2 tbsp chopped fresh cilantro

2 tbsp chopped fresh parsley

¼ cup (60 ml) olive oil

Seasoning to taste

18 endive leaves

Cilantro, coarsely chopped, for garnish

Lemon wedges

METHOD

In a bowl, mix salmon, egg yolks, mustard, maple syrup, lemon juice, green onions, chives, cilantro and parsley.

Slowly add olive oil and mix. Season to taste.

Divide mixture among endive leaves. Garnish with cilantro and serve with lemon wedges.

Serve with raw vegetables.

Nutrition Facts Per serving	
Amount	% Daily Value
Calories 340	
Fat 20 g	31%
Saturated 3.5 g	
+ Trans 0 g	
Polyunsaturated 4 g	
Omega-6 1 g	
Omega-3 2.5 g	
Monounsaturated 4 g	
Cholesterol 140 mg	48%
Sodium 330 mg	14%
Potassium 1030 mg	29%
Carbohydrates 7 g	2%
Fiber 3 g	12%
Sugar 3 g	
Protein 33 g	
Vitamin A 255 ER	25%
Vitamin C 15 mg	25%
Calcium 93 mg	8%
Iron 2.8 mg	20%
Phosphorus 352.2 mg	30%

DID YOU KNOW?

Wild salmon feed off small crustaceans. These crustaceans contain carotenoids that give salmon that pink to bright red color it's known for. Farmed salmon are fed pellets that contain synthetic coloring to help obtain that pinkish hue.

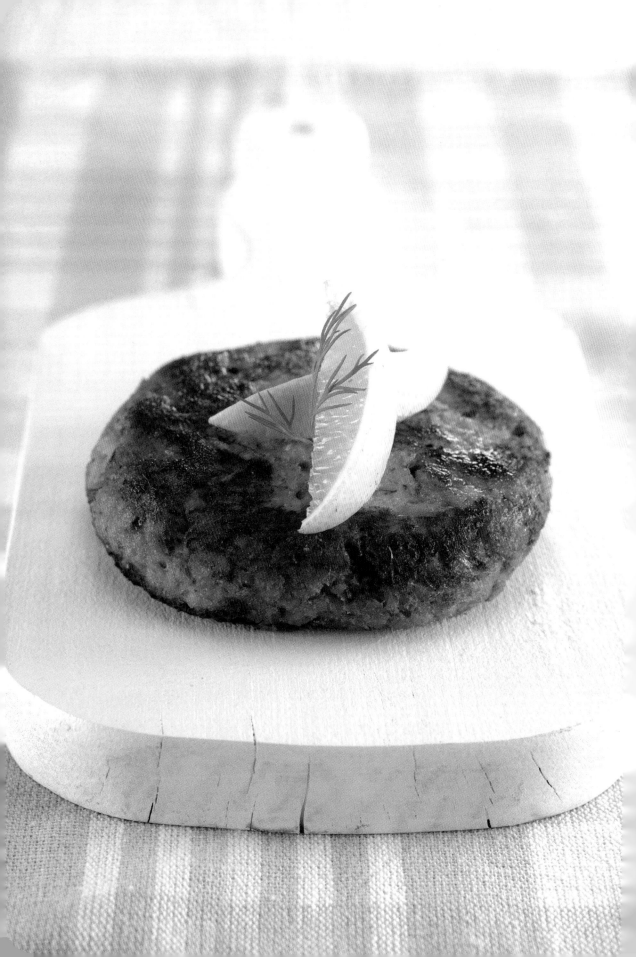

OMEGA
PATTIES

4 SERVINGS
15 MINUTES
30 MINUTES

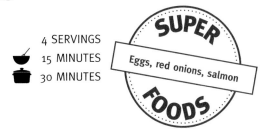

SUPER
FOODS

Eggs, red onions, salmon

INGREDIENTS

2 sweet potatoes, peeled and cubed

1 small **red onion**, minced

2 cans (each 7.5 oz/213 g) **salmon**, drained and flaked

1 **egg**, beaten

1 tbsp Dijon mustard

1 tbsp chopped fresh dill

Leaves of 1 sprig fresh thyme

Tabasco to taste

Seasoning to taste

1 tbsp olive oil

1 lemon, cut in wedges

METHOD

In a saucepan over medium-high heat, cook sweet potatoes in boiling water for about 20 minutes or until tender. Drain and mash potatoes.

Meanwhile, in a bowl, combine onion, salmon, egg, mustard, dill, thyme and Tabasco. Add potatoes and season to taste.

Using your hands, shape mixture into 8 patties, ¾ inch (2 cm) thick.

In a skillet, heat oil over medium heat. Place patties in skillet and cook for 5 minutes on each side.

Serve with lemon wedges.

COMMON MISCONCEPTIONS

Salmon is a fatty fish.

TRUE, however . . . even though salmon is considered one of the fattiest fish, its fat content is similar to that of lean meat. Plus, the fat in salmon is actually good for your health.

Nutrition Facts Per serving	
Amount	**% Daily Value**
Calories 240	
Fat 11 g	17%
Saturated 2 g	
+ Trans 0 g	
Polyunsaturated 2.5 g	
Omega-6 0.4 g	
Omega-3 1.5 g	
Monounsaturated 3 g	
Cholesterol 65 mg	22%
Sodium 480 mg	20%
Potassium 610 mg	17%
Carbohydrates 19 g	6%
Fiber 3 g	12%
Sugar 5 g	
Protein 17 g	
Vitamin A 962 ER	100%
Vitamin C 17 mg	30%
Calcium 221 mg	20%
Iron 1.9 mg	15%
Phosphorus 928.5 mg	80%

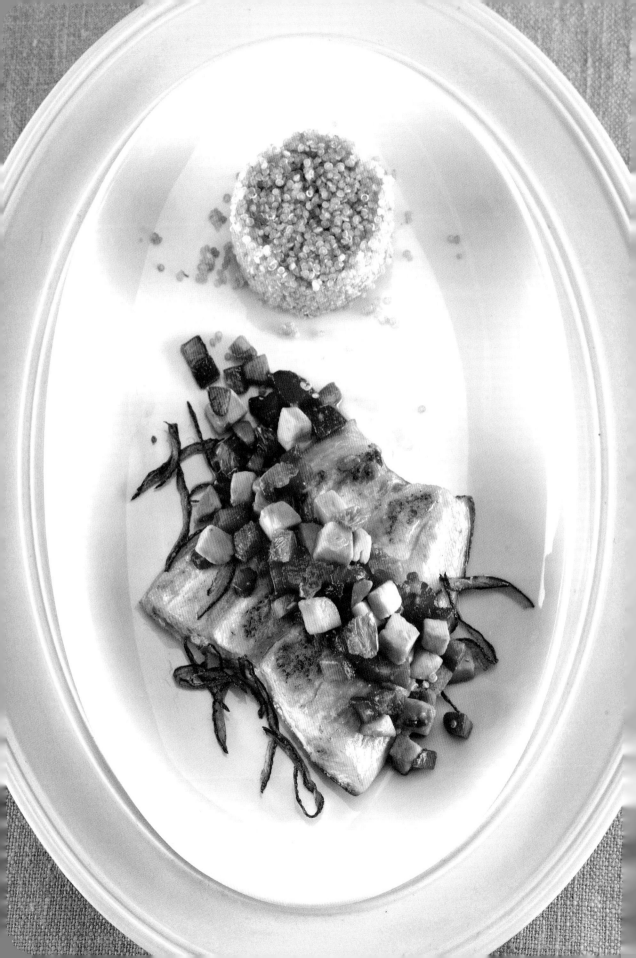

SALMON WITH AVOCADO, GRAPEFRUIT
AND STRAWBERRY SALSA

4 SERVINGS
15 MINUTES
10 MINUTES

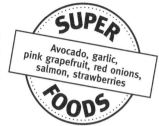

SUPER FOODS

Avocado, garlic, pink grapefruit, red onions, salmon, strawberries

INGREDIENTS

1 tbsp olive oil

1 small **red onion**, minced

1 clove **garlic**, minced

4 **salmon** filets
(each 4 oz/120 g),
skin on

1 **avocado**, diced

1 small **pink grapefruit**, diced

15 **strawberries**, diced

Pinch crushed hot pepper flakes

Juice of ½ lemon

METHOD

In a skillet, heat oil over high heat and sauté onion and garlic for 3 minutes. Reduce heat to medium and cook salmon for 8 to 10 minutes, depending on thickness.

Meanwhile, in a bowl, combine avocado, grapefruit, strawberries and hot pepper flakes. Drizzle with lemon juice and mix well.

Top salmon with salsa.

Serve with rice or quinoa.

── CHEF'S TIPS ──

- Wrap avocado in newspaper to help accelerate the ripening process.
- Roll avocado in your hands a few minutes for easier peeling.
- Once peeled, drizzle avocado with lemon or lime juice to halt the oxidation process and prevent it from going black.

Nutrition Facts Per serving		
Amount		% Daily Value
Calories 380		
Fat 25 g		38%
Saturated 4.5 g		
+ Trans 0 g		
Polyunsaturated 6 g		
Omega-6 3 g		
Omega-3 2.5 g		
Monounsaturated 10 g		
Cholesterol 70 mg		23%
Sodium 75 mg		3%
Potassium 800 mg		23%
Carbohydrates 12 g		4%
Fiber 5 g		20%
Sugar 3 g		
Protein 27 g		
Vitamin A 25 ER		2%
Vitamin C 30 mg		50%
Calcium 46 mg		4%
Iron 1 mg		6%
Phosphorus 337.9 mg		30%

MAPLE-AND-MUSTARD-CRUSTED
SALMON

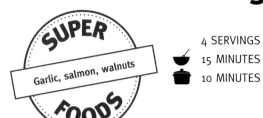

SUPER FOODS

Garlic, salmon, walnuts

4 SERVINGS

15 MINUTES

10 MINUTES

INGREDIENTS

¼ cup (60 ml) olive oil

2 tbsp Dijon mustard

2 tbsp balsamic vinegar

1 tbsp mayonnaise

1 tbsp maple syrup

3 cloves **garlic,** minced

1 cup (250 ml) chopped **walnuts**

2 tbsp chopped fresh cilantro

2 tbsp chopped fresh parsley

1 sprig fresh rosemary

Seasoning to taste

4 **salmon** filets (each 4 oz/120 g)

¼ cup (60 ml) fresh cilantro, for garnish

METHOD

Position rack in center of oven and preheat to 425°F (220°C). Line a baking sheet with parchment paper.

In a bowl, combine all ingredients except for the salmon and cilantro for garnish. On prepared baking sheet, place salmon filets and brush with olive oil mixture. Cook in center of preheated oven for about 10 minutes, depending on thickness.

Garnish with cilantro prior to serving.

Serve with vegetables.

Nutrition Facts Per serving	
Amount	**% Daily Value**
Calories 510	
Fat 37 g	57%
Saturated 5 g + Trans 0 g	
Polyunsaturated 21 g	
Omega-6 15 g	
Omega-3 5 g	
Monounsaturated 8 g	
Cholesterol 75 mg	25%
Sodium 180 mg	8%
Potassium 690 mg	20%
Carbohydrates 12 g	4%
Fiber 3 g	12%
Sugar 5 g	
Protein 31 g	
Vitamin A 56 ER	6%
Vitamin C 17 mg	30%
Calcium 89 mg	8%
Iron 2.4 mg	15%
Phosphorus 409.2 mg	35%

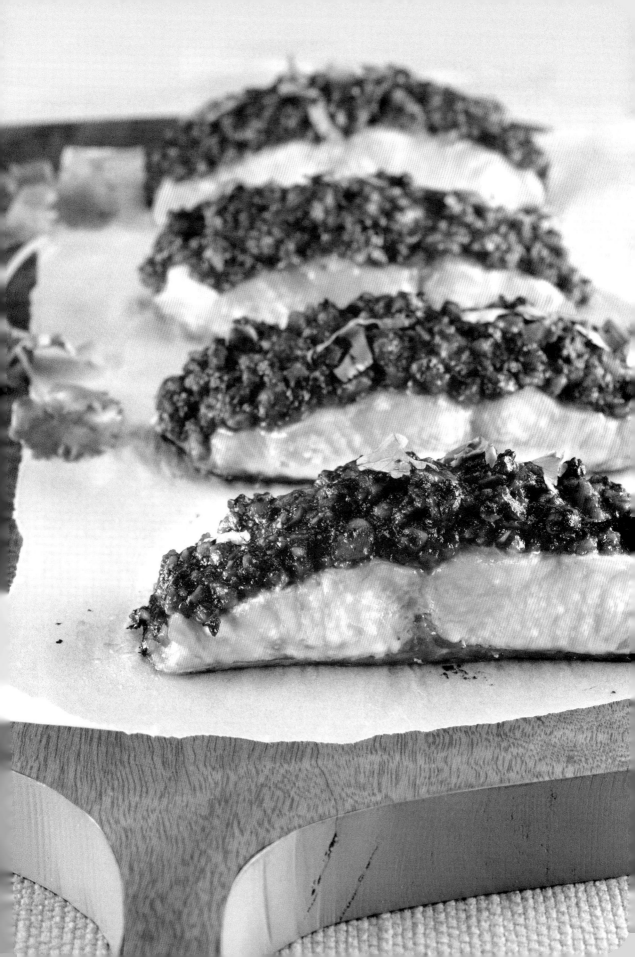

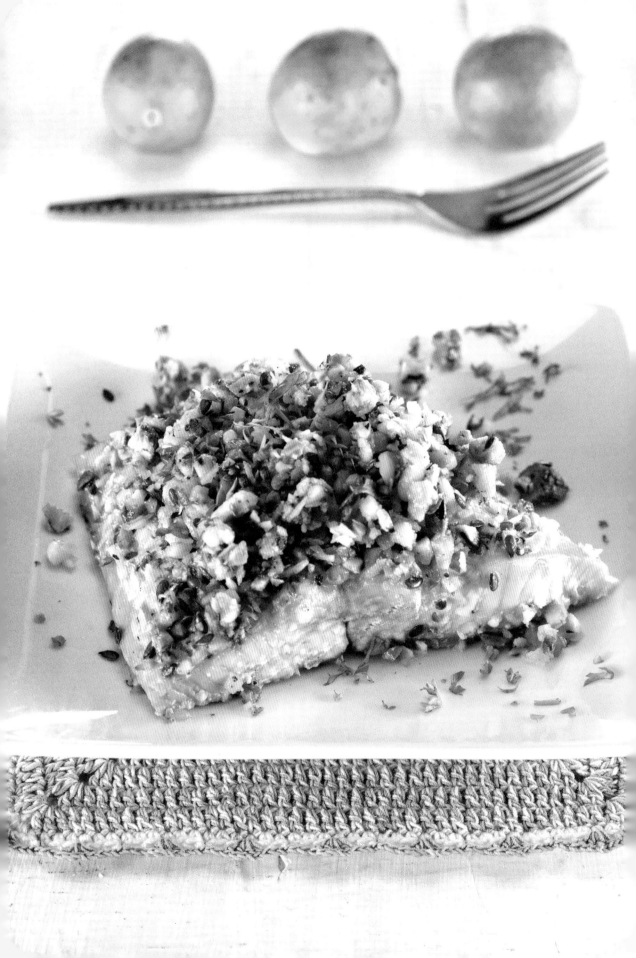

COCONUT, WALNUT AND PISTACHIO
SALMON

4 SERVINGS

20 MINUTES

10 MINUTES

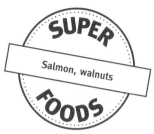

Salmon, walnuts

SUPER FOODS

INGREDIENTS

¼ cup (60 ml) chopped pistachios

¼ cup (60 ml) chopped **walnuts**

¼ cup (60 ml) grated coconut

2 tbsp olive oil

1 tbsp chia seeds or ground flaxseeds

3 tbsp chopped fresh basil

2 tsp grated Parmesan

Seasoning to taste

4 **salmon** filets (each 4 oz/120 g)

Juice of 1 lime

¼ cup (60 ml) chopped fresh parsley

METHOD

Position rack in center of oven and preheat to 350°F (180°C). Line a baking sheet with parchment paper.

In a bowl, combine all ingredients, except salmon, lime juice and parsley.

Place salmon filets on prepared baking sheet and top with prepared mixture. Cook in center of preheated oven for about 8 minutes, depending on thickness.

Before serving, drizzle with lime juice and garnish with parsley.

Nutrition Facts Per serving	
Amount	% Daily Value
Calories 430	
Fat 32 g	49%
Saturated 7 g	
+ Trans 0 g	
Polyunsaturated 10 g	
Omega-6 6 g	
Omega-3 3.5 g	
Monounsaturated 8 g	
Cholesterol 70 mg	23%
Sodium 90 mg	4%
Potassium 620 mg	18%
Carbohydrates 7 g	2%
Fiber 3 g	12%
Sugar 1 g	
Protein 29 g	
Vitamin A 68 ER	6%
Vitamin C 12 mg	20%
Calcium 73 mg	6%
Iron 1.8 mg	15%
Phosphorus 399.1 mg	35%

DID YOU KNOW?

The omega-3s found in salmon come from the algae they eat.

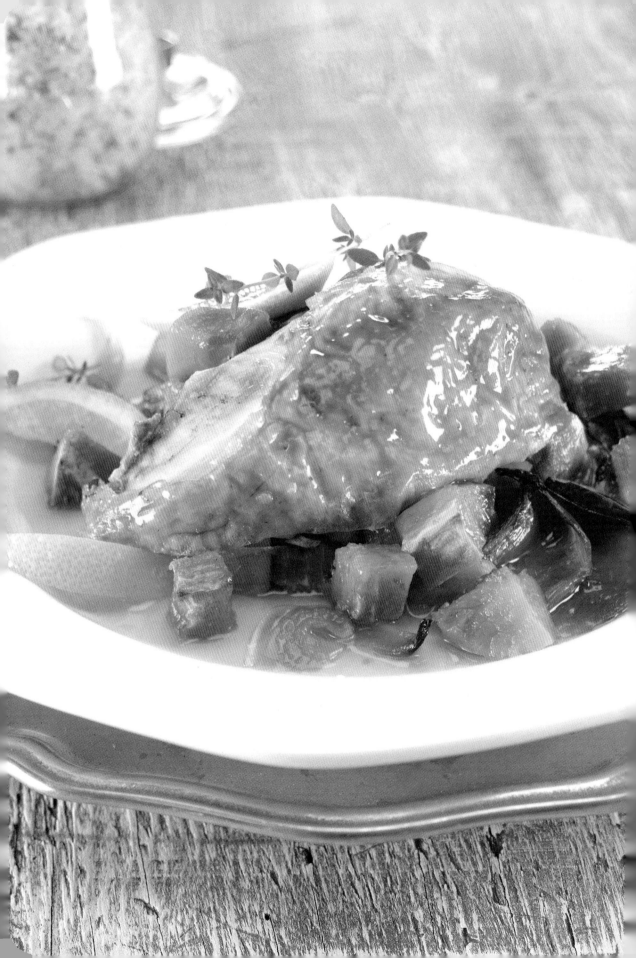

ROAST CHICKEN WITH LEMON
AND THYME

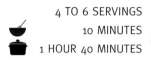

4 TO 6 SERVINGS
10 MINUTES
1 HOUR 40 MINUTES

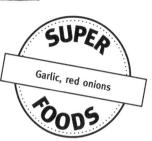

Garlic, red onions

INGREDIENTS

1 whole chicken
(2 to 3 lbs/1 to 1.5 kg)

2 lemons, cut in wedges

3 sprigs fresh thyme

5 cloves **garlic,** halved

1 tbsp olive oil

3 sprigs fresh rosemary

3 sweet potatoes, cubed

2 stalks celery, sliced
on the diagonal

2 **red onions,** cut in eighths

Seasoning to taste

1 lemon, cut in wedges,
for serving

METHOD

Position rack in center of oven and preheat to 350°F (180°C).

Stuff chicken with lemon wedges, thyme and garlic. Truss the bird and place in a large cooking dish.

In a bowl, combine oil, rosemary, sweet potatoes, celery and onions. Season to taste and spread mixture around chicken. Cook in center of preheated oven for about 1 hour and 40 minutes until the juices run clear.

Empty stuffing and carve chicken.

Serve immediately with sweet potato mixture and lemon wedges.

Nutrition Facts		
Per serving (⅙ of recipe)		
Amount		% Daily Value
Calories 610		
Fat 31 g		48%
Saturated 8 g		
+ Trans 0 g		
Polyunsaturated 6 g		
Omega-6 6 g		
Omega-3 0.4 g		
Monounsaturated 11 g		
Cholesterol 160 mg		53%
Sodium 210 mg		9%
Potassium 940 mg		27%
Carbohydrates 30 g		10%
Fiber 5 g		20%
Sugar 7 g		
Protein 53 g		
Vitamin A 996 ER		100%
Vitamin C 37 mg		60%
Calcium 121 mg		10%
Iron 4.1 mg		30%
Phosphorus 462 mg		40%

COCONUT MILK, QUINOA AND RED PEPPER
CHICKEN

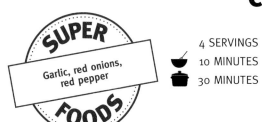

SUPER FOODS

Garlic, red onions, red pepper

4 SERVINGS
10 MINUTES
30 MINUTES

INGREDIENTS

1 tbsp olive oil

1 lb (454 g) chicken breasts

1 small **red onion**, finely chopped

2 **red peppers**, diced

1 green pepper, diced

6 cloves **garlic**, minced

2 tsp cumin seeds

1 tsp paprika

1 tsp curry powder

½ cup (125 ml) coconut milk

Seasoning to taste

1½ cups (375 ml) low-sodium chicken broth

¾ cup (180 ml) quinoa, rinsed and strained

Parsley, for garnish

METHOD

In a skillet, heat oil over medium heat and brown chicken breasts for 4 minutes each side. Add onion, peppers, garlic, cumin, paprika and curry. Cook for about 10 minutes. Pour coconut milk into skillet and continue cooking a few minutes. Season to taste.

Meanwhile, in a saucepan over medium heat, bring broth to a boil and add quinoa. Reduce heat to low. Cover and let simmer for 12 minutes. Drain.

Serve chicken with quinoa and garnish with parsley.

Nutrition Facts Per serving	
Amount	**% Daily Value**
Calories 330	
Fat 12 g	18%
Saturated 2.5 g	
+ Trans 0 g	
Polyunsaturated 2 g	
Omega-6 2 g	
Omega-3 0.2 g	
Monounsaturated 3.5 g	
Cholesterol 85 mg	28%
Sodium 135 mg	6%
Potassium 770 mg	22%
Carbohydrates 23 g	8%
Fiber 3 g	12%
Sugar 6 g	
Protein 33 g	
Vitamin A 186 ER	20%
Vitamin C 119 mg	200%
Calcium 135 mg	10%
Iron 4.8 mg	35%
Phosphorus 326.7 mg	30%

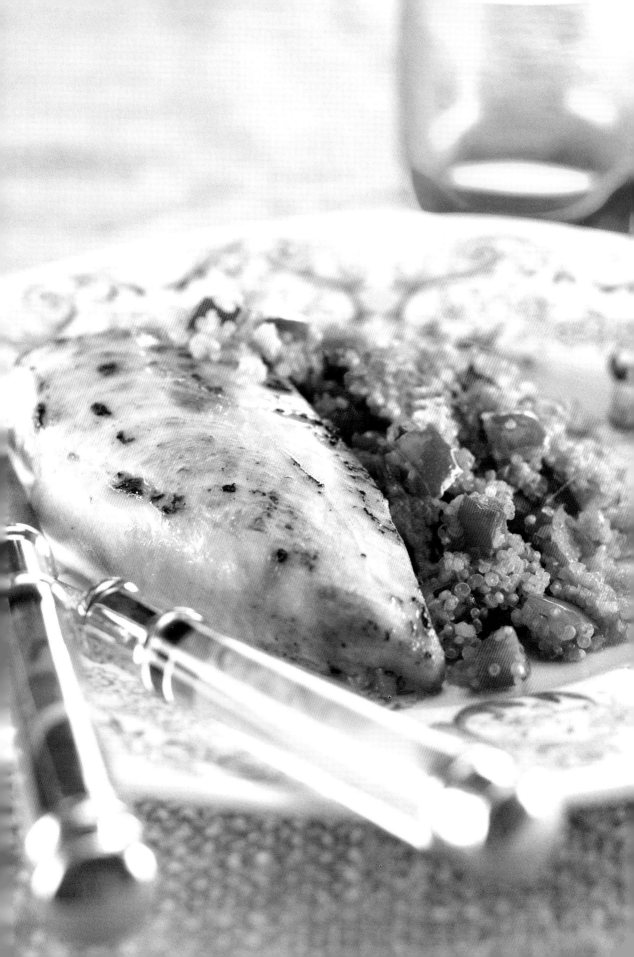

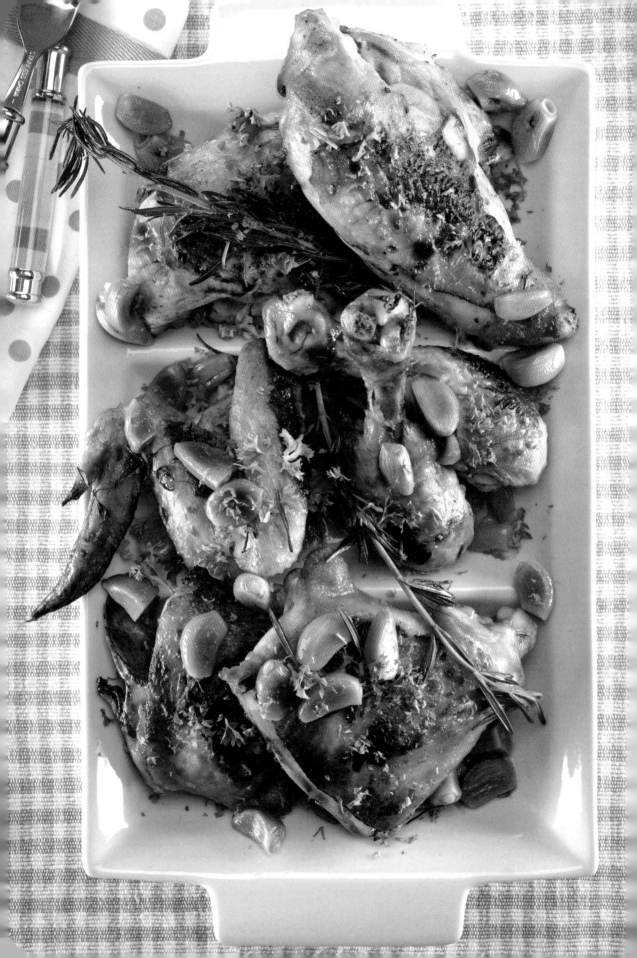

CHICKEN WITH
50 CLOVES OF GARLIC

6 SERVINGS
20 MINUTES
1 HOUR

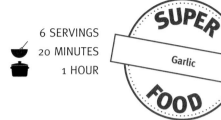

SUPER
Garlic
FOOD

INGREDIENTS

3½ lbs (1.6 kg) chicken, cut in pieces

2 tsp Dijon mustard

Seasoning to taste

2 tbsp olive oil

1½ cups (375 ml) white wine

50 cloves **garlic**, peeled

3 sprigs fresh thyme

2 sprigs fresh rosemary

½ cup (125 ml) chopped fresh parsley, for garnish

METHOD

Preheat oven to 350°F (180°C).

Brush chicken with mustard and season to taste.

In a large ovenproof skillet, heat oil over medium-high heat and brown chicken for 5 minutes or until sides are golden. Remove chicken from skillet.

In same skillet, add white wine, garlic, thyme and rosemary, stirring constantly. Return chicken to skillet.

Cover and cook in preheated oven for 1 hour. Add water, if needed.

Garnish with parsley prior to serving.

Nutrition Facts Per serving	
Amount	**% Daily Value**
Calories 516	
Fat 16 g	25%
Saturated 11 g	
+ Trans 0 g	
Polyunsaturated 8 g	
Omega-6 8 g	
Omega-3 0.5 g	
Monounsaturated 14 g	
Cholesterol 200 mg	68%
Sodium 250 mg	11%
Potassium 1460 mg	42%
Carbohydrates 68 g	23%
Fiber 5 g	20%
Sugar 2 g	
Protein 25 g	
Vitamin A 125 ER	10%
Vitamin C 72 mg	120%
Calcium 418 mg	40%
Iron 7.7 mg	50%
Phosphorus 797.6 mg	70%

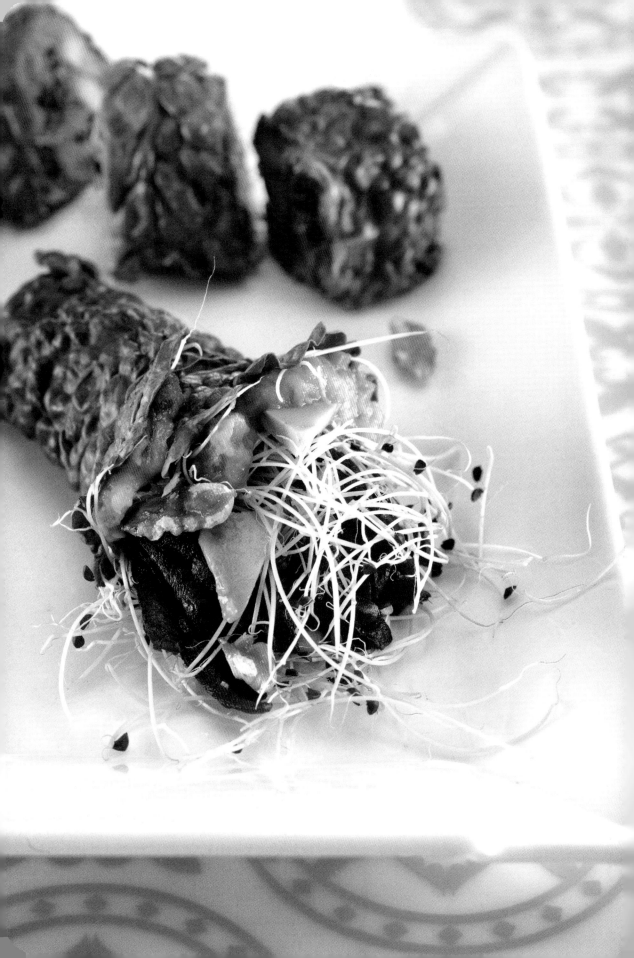

LIMA BEAN
WRAPS

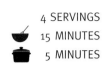

4 SERVINGS
15 MINUTES
5 MINUTES

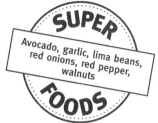

Avocado, garlic, lima beans, red onions, red pepper, walnuts

INGREDIENTS

For the lima bean purée

2 tbsp olive oil

1 small **red onion**, finely minced

3 to 5 cloves **garlic**, minced

1 **red pepper**, thinly sliced

1 can (19 oz/540 ml) **lima beans**, drained and rinsed

Juice of ½ lemon

3 tbsp chopped fresh parsley

Thyme and sage, to taste

Salt, pepper and paprika, to taste

For the wraps

8 collard green leaves, blanched 15 seconds in boiling water

1 beet or 1 carrot, grated

¼ cup (60 ml) alfalfa sprouts

1 **avocado**, sliced

2 tbsp crushed **walnuts**

METHOD

In a skillet, heat oil over high heat and sauté onion, garlic and pepper for about 5 minutes. Let cool for 5 minutes.

Add lima beans, lemon juice, parsley, herbs and seasonings. Transfer to a blender and purée. Add water until desired consistency.

Divide mixture among collard green leaves. Add beets, alfalfa sprouts, avocado and walnuts. Tuck ends inward and roll.

Nutrition Facts Per serving	
Amount	**% Daily Value**
Calories 320	
Fat 16 g	25%
Saturated 2 g + Trans 0 g	
Polyunsaturated 2.5 g	
Omega-6 2 g	
Omega-3 0.4 g	
Monounsaturated 5 g	
Cholesterol 0 mg	0%
Sodium 25 mg	0%
Potassium 900 mg	26%
Carbohydrates 36 g	12%
Fiber 9 g	36%
Sugar 5 g	
Protein 9 g	
Vitamin A 130 ER	15%
Vitamin C 62 mg	100%
Calcium 92 mg	8%
Iron 3 mg	20%
Phosphorus 187.2 mg	15%

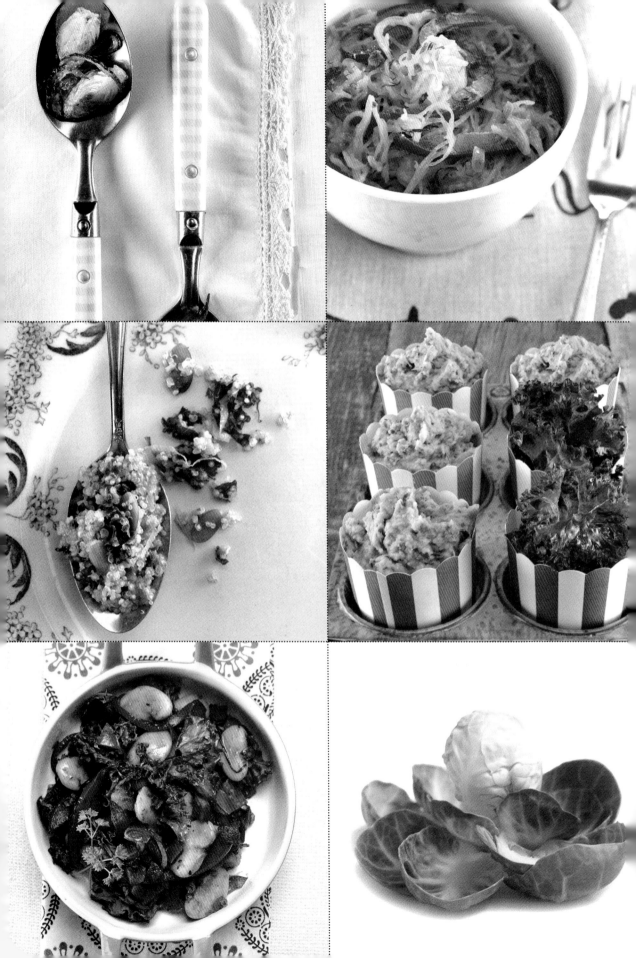

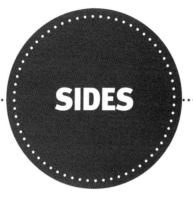

SIDES

GINGER
BRUSSELS SPROUTS

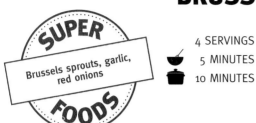

SUPER FOODS

Brussels sprouts, garlic, red onions

4 SERVINGS

5 MINUTES

10 MINUTES

INGREDIENTS

1 tbsp olive oil

1 small **red onion**, minced

2 cloves **garlic**, minced

2 cups (500 ml) **Brussels sprouts**, halved or quartered

1 tbsp minced fresh ginger

METHOD

In a skillet, heat oil over medium heat and sauté onion, garlic and Brussels sprouts for 5 minutes.

Add ginger and continue cooking for 3 minutes.

Nutrition Facts Per serving	
Amount	**% Daily Value**
Calories 90	
Fat 3.5 g	5%
Saturated 0.5 g	
+ Trans 0 g	
Polyunsaturated 0.1 g	
Omega-6 0.1 g	
Omega-3 0.1 g	
Monounsaturated 0 g	
Cholesterol 0 mg	0%
Sodium 15 mg	1%
Potassium 280 mg	8%
Carbohydrates 12 g	4%
Fiber 3 g	12%
Sugar 3 g	
Protein 3 g	
Vitamin A 34 ER	4%
Vitamin C 44 mg	70%
Calcium 49 mg	4%
Iron 0.9 mg	6%
Phosphorus 60 mg	6%

──── DID YOU KNOW? ────

Brussels sprouts contain several classes of goitrogens, which have an impact on thyroid function. However, they become inactive when heated and do not affect the thyroid gland of healthy individuals.

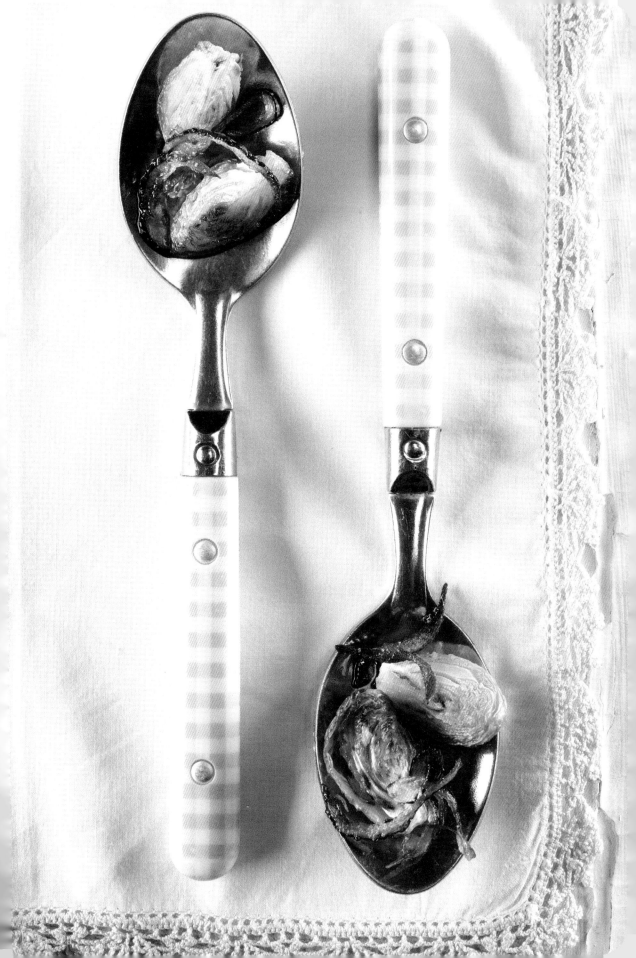

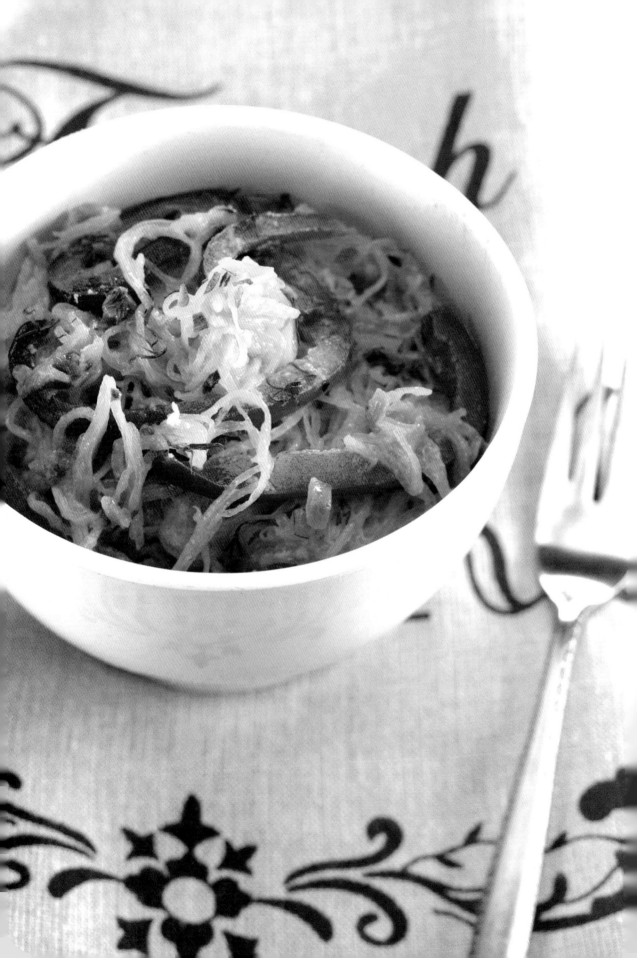

SPAGHETTI SQUASH WITH RED PEPPERS
AND GOAT CHEESE

4 SERVINGS
15 MINUTES
45 MINUTES

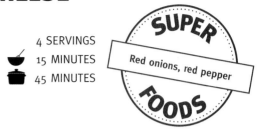

Red onions, red pepper

INGREDIENTS

1 large spaghetti squash

1 tsp ground turmeric

2 tbsp olive oil

1 small **red onion**, minced

1 **red pepper**, thinly sliced

½ tsp crushed hot pepper flakes (optional)

1½ cups (375 ml) low-sodium vegetable broth

1 tsp lemon zest

3 tbsp lemon juice

2 tbsp finely chopped fresh dill

¼ cup (60 ml) soft goat cheese

Seasoning to taste

METHOD

Position rack in center of oven and preheat to 375°F (190°C).

Cut squash in half and remove seeds. Place squash on a baking sheet, cut-side down. Brush with oil. Cook in center of preheated oven for 30 to 40 minutes or until flesh is easily pierced with a knife. Let cool at room temperature for a few minutes.

Using a fork, gently scrape out "spaghetti" strands. Place in a bowl and add turmeric. Set aside.

In a skillet, heat oil over medium heat and sauté onion, pepper and pepper flakes, if using, for a few minutes. Add broth and lemon zest. Reduce by one quarter.

Add lemon juice and dill. Add cheese. Stir until melted. Remove from heat, add spaghetti squash and season to taste. Serve immediately.

Nutrition Facts Per serving	
Amount	% Daily Value
Calories 330	
Fat 12 g	18%
Saturated 4 g	
+ Trans 0 g	
Polyunsaturated 1 g	
Omega-6 0.5 g	
Omega-3 0.4 g	
Monounsaturated 1 g	
Cholesterol 10 mg	3%
Sodium 210 mg	9%
Potassium 1030 mg	29%
Carbohydrates 48 g	16%
Fiber 9 g	36%
Sugar 20 g	
Protein 8 g	
Vitamin A 882 ER	90%
Vitamin C 72 mg	120%
Calcium 264 mg	25%
Iron 2.9 mg	20%
Phosphorus 196.5 mg	20%

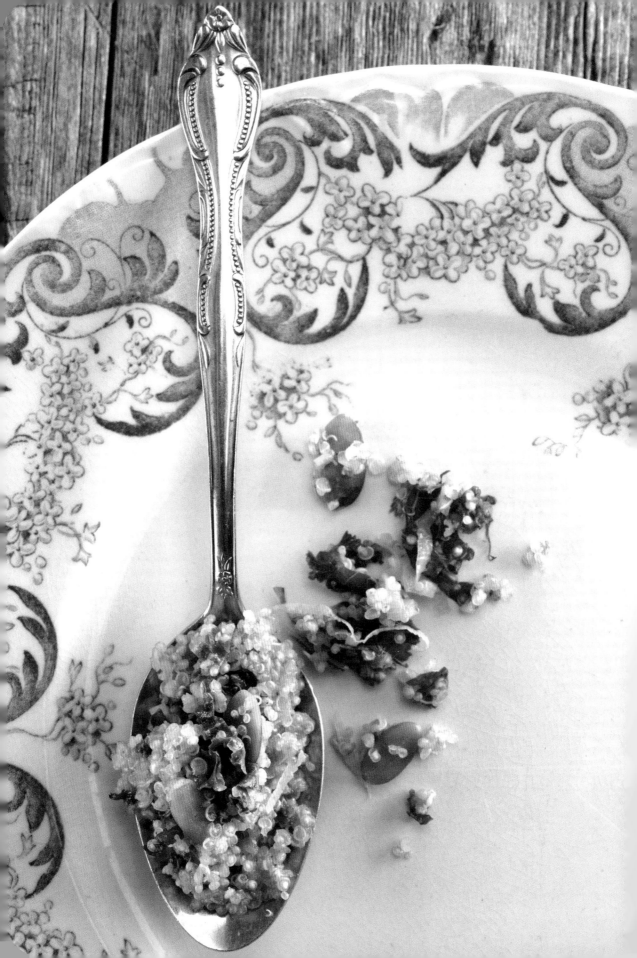

QUINOA AND KALE
PILAF

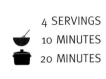

4 SERVINGS
10 MINUTES
20 MINUTES

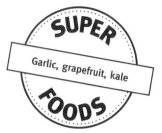

Garlic, grapefruit, kale

INGREDIENTS

1 tbsp olive oil

¼ leek, white part only, minced

2 cloves **garlic**, minced

3 cups (750 ml) vegetable or chicken broth

1 cup (250 ml) quinoa, rinsed and drained

¼ cup (60 ml) toasted pumpkin seeds

½ cup (125 ml) chopped fresh parsley

1 sprig fresh thyme

2 tbsp **grapefruit** juice

2 tsp lemon zest

Seasoning to taste

2 cups (500 ml) coarsely chopped **kale**, stems removed

METHOD

In a skillet, heat oil over medium heat and sauté leek, stirring occasionally, for about 3 minutes or until golden.

Add remaining ingredients, except for kale, and continue cooking over medium heat for 15 minutes.

Add kale in the last 5 minutes of cooking. Remove thyme sprig.

Nutrition Facts Per serving	
Amount	% Daily Value
Calories 420	
Fat 11 g	17%
Saturated 1.5 g	
+ Trans 0 g	
Polyunsaturated 3 g	
Omega-6 3 g	
Omega-3 0.1 g	
Monounsaturated 2 g	
Cholesterol 0 mg	0%
Sodium 200 mg	8%
Potassium 1290 mg	37%
Carbohydrates 67 g	64%
Fiber 16 g	64%
Sugar 13 g	
Protein 14 g	
Vitamin A 1736 ER	170%
Vitamin C 119 mg	200%
Calcium 303 mg	30%
Iron 8.1 mg	60%
Phosphorus 395.2 mg	35%

LIMA BEAN AND
CARAMELIZED ONION PURÉE

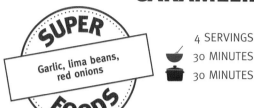

🥄 4 SERVINGS
🥄 30 MINUTES
🍲 30 MINUTES

INGREDIENTS

2 cans (each 19 oz/540 ml) **lima beans**, drained and rinsed

Juice of 1 lemon

¼ cup (60 ml) chopped fresh parsley

¼ cup (60 ml) chopped fresh cilantro

For the caramelized onions

3 tbsp olive oil

2 **red onions**, sliced

1 clove **garlic**

1 tsp whole cumin seeds

Seasoning to taste

METHOD

In a skillet, heat oil over medium-high heat and caramelize onions and garlic, stirring constantly, for about 20 minutes. Reduce heat to medium and continue cooking another 5 minutes or until onions are thoroughly caramelized. (Add water if onions stick to skillet.) Add cumin and season to taste.

In a food processor, purée lima beans. Add caramelized onions, lemon juice, parsley and cilantro. Mix until slightly lumpy texture is obtained. Season to taste.

Serve with Kale Chips (see p. 85).

Nutrition Facts Per serving	
Amount	**% Daily Value**
Calories 340	
Fat 11 g	17%
Saturated 1.5 g	
+ Trans 0 g	
Polyunsaturated 0.3 g	
Omega-6 0.2 g	
Omega-3 0.1 g	
Monounsaturated 0.2 g	
Cholesterol 0 mg	0%
Sodium 40 mg	2%
Potassium 1190 mg	34%
Carbohydrates 48 g	16%
Fiber 10 g	40%
Sugar 6 g	
Protein 12 g	
Vitamin A 110 ER	10%
Vitamin C 49 mg	80%
Calcium 132 mg	10%
Iron 6.1 mg	45%
Phosphorus 247.3 mg	20%

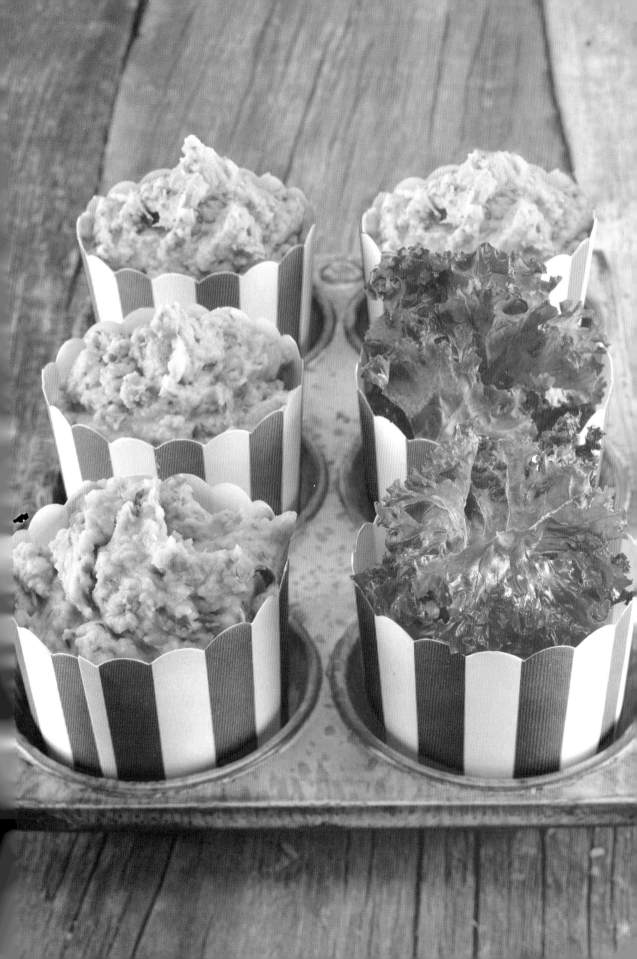

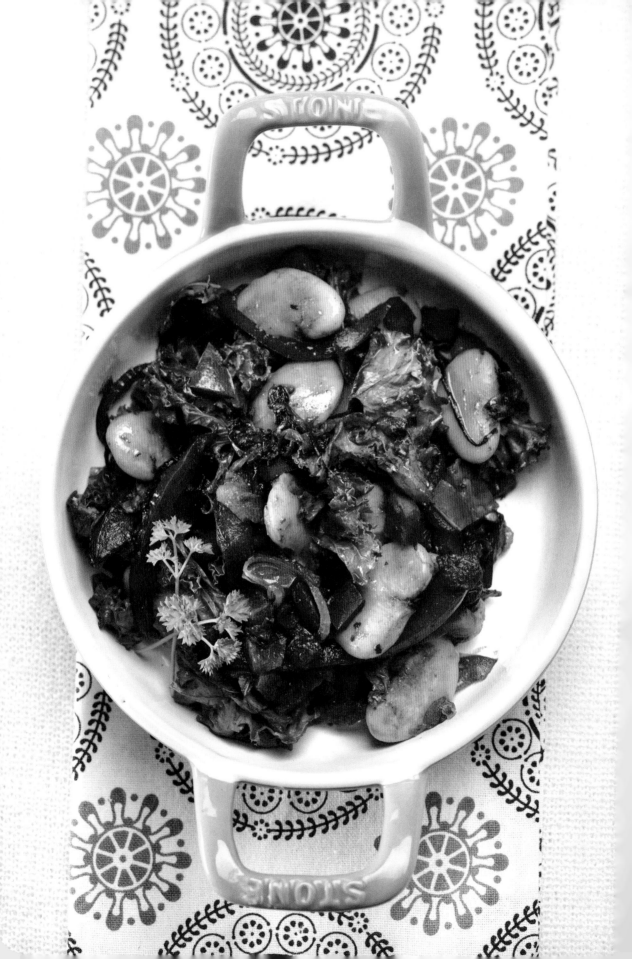

LIMA BEANS WITH
TOMATOES AND SAGE

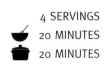

4 SERVINGS
20 MINUTES
20 MINUTES

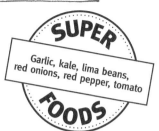

SUPER FOODS

Garlic, kale, lima beans, red onions, red pepper, tomato

INGREDIENTS

1 tbsp olive oil

1 small **red onion**, minced

5 cloves **garlic**, minced

1 **red pepper**, thinly sliced

2 cups (500 ml) shredded **kale**, stems removed

1 can (19 oz/540 ml) giant **lima beans**, drained and rinsed

5 fresh **tomatoes**, diced

2 tbsp finely chopped fresh parsley

4 tsp finely chopped fresh sage

Seasoning to taste

2 tbsp miso

2 tbsp fresh parsley, for garnish

METHOD

In a large skillet, heat oil over medium heat and sauté onion, garlic, pepper and kale for 5 minutes. Add remaining ingredients, except for miso and parsley for garnish. Cover and continue to cook for 15 minutes.

Just before serving, add miso and stir well. Garnish with parsley.

LIMA BEANS AND FLATULENCE

The high levels of oligosaccharides (a sort of carbohydrate) found in lima beans are largely responsible for the gassiness you feel after eating them. To lower these sugar levels, we recommend quickly soaking lima beans before consuming them. In addition to cutting down on cooking time, soaking beans makes them more digestible. The easiest way to soak lima beans is to place them in a large saucepan of cold water. Place the pot over medium-high heat and bring to a boil. Let simmer for 1 to 2 minutes. Remove from heat and let sit for 1 hour. Rinse beans under cold water prior to cooking. (The soaking water is not fit for consumption.) It's recommended to thoroughly rinse canned beans prior to consuming them.

Nutrition Facts Per serving	
Amount	% Daily Value
Calories 260	
Fat 5 g	8%
Saturated 1 g	
+ Trans 0 g	
Polyunsaturated 1 g	
Omega-6 0.5 g	
Omega-3 0.1 g	
Monounsaturated 0.2 g	
Cholesterol 0 mg	0%
Sodium 320 mg	13%
Potassium 1110 mg	32%
Carbohydrates 43 g	14%
Fiber 9 g	36%
Sugar 9 g	
Protein 11 g	
Vitamin A 484 ER	50%
Vitamin C 92 mg	150%
Calcium 175 mg	15%
Iron 3.6 mg	25%
Phosphorus 213.5 mg	20%

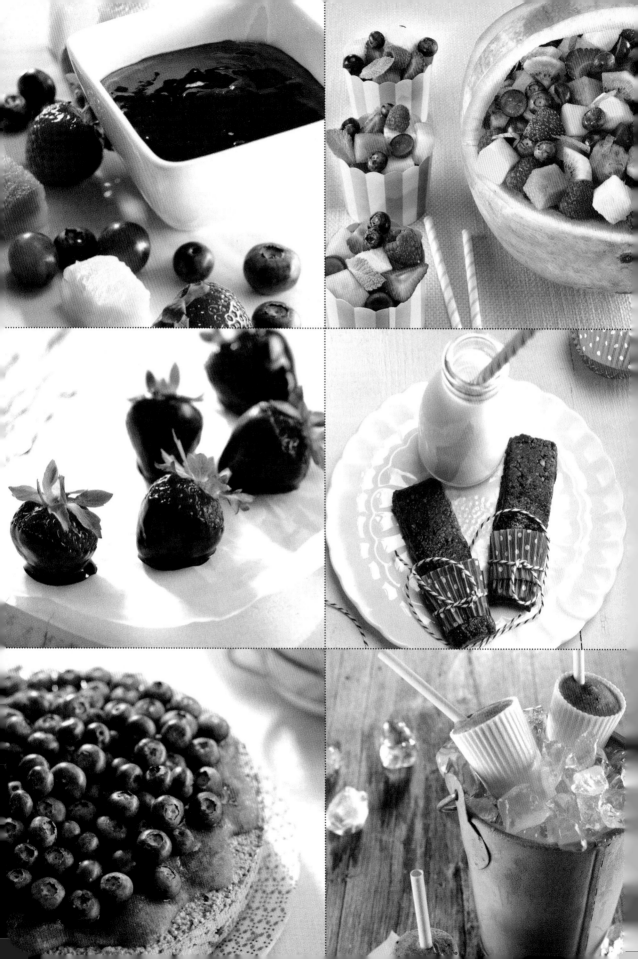

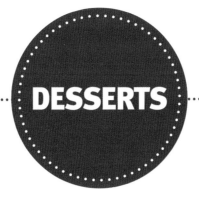

DESSERTS

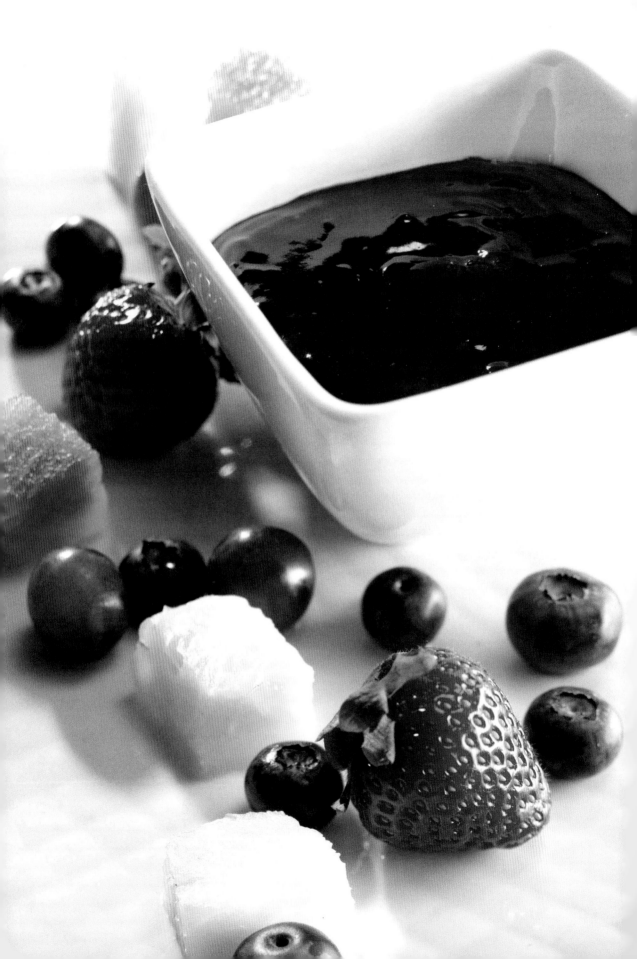

FRUITY CHOCOLATE
FONDUE

6 SERVINGS

20 MINUTES

10 MINUTES

Blueberries, red grapes, strawberries

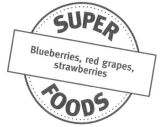

INGREDIENTS

2 cups (500 ml) assorted fruit
(**red grapes, blueberries, strawberries**, melons, pineapple), cut in cubes

1 cup (250 ml) chocolate chips (70% cacao)

¼ cup (60 ml) date purée
or ¼ cup (60 ml) maple syrup

METHOD

Arrange fruit on serving platter.

In a fondue pot on very low heat, melt chocolate. Add date purée and mix well.

Spear fruit with fondue forks and dip in chocolate.

Nutrition Facts Per serving	
Amount	**% Daily Value**
Calories 270	
Fat 7 g	11%
Saturated 4 g	
+ Trans 0 g	
Polyunsaturated 0.1 g	
Omega-6 0 g	
Omega-3 0 g	
Monounsaturated 0.5 g	
Cholesterol 0 mg	0%
Sodium 5 mg	0%
Potassium 110 mg	3%
Carbohydrates 49 g	16%
Fiber 3 g	12%
Sugar 39 g	
Protein 2 g	
Vitamin A 3 ER	0%
Vitamin C 8 mg	15%
Calcium 17 mg	2%
Iron 0.9 mg	6%
Phosphorus 10.6 mg	0%

BERRIES IN RED WINE
— WITH SPICES —

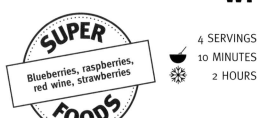

SUPER
FOODS

Blueberries, raspberries,
red wine, strawberries

🥣 4 SERVINGS

10 MINUTES

❄ 2 HOURS

INGREDIENTS

1½ cups (375 ml) **red wine**

¼ cup (60 ml) maple syrup

2 cloves (optional)

1 cinnamon stick

Juice of 1 orange

Juice of 1 lemon

1 tbsp water

2 cups (500 ml) **strawberries,**
halved

1 cup (250 ml) **raspberries**

1 cup (250 ml) **blueberries**

1 tbsp chopped fresh peppermint

METHOD

In a large bowl, combine red wine, maple syrup, cloves, if using, cinnamon, orange juice, lemon juice and water. Add berries and mint.

Refrigerate for at least 2 hours.

Serve in martini glasses.

Nutrition Facts Per serving	
Amount	**% Daily Value**
Calories 160	
Fat 1 g	2%
Saturated 0.1 g	
+ Trans 0 g	
Polyunsaturated 0.4 g	
Omega-6 0.3 g	
Omega-3 0.2 g	
Monounsaturated 0.1 g	
Cholesterol 0 mg	0%
Sodium 10 mg	0%
Potassium 420 mg	12%
Carbohydrates 36 g	12%
Fiber 6 g	24%
Sugar 23 g	
Protein 2 g	
Vitamin A 14 ER	2%
Vitamin C 77 mg	130%
Calcium 70 mg	6%
Iron 1.9 mg	15%
Phosphorus 54.4 mg	4%

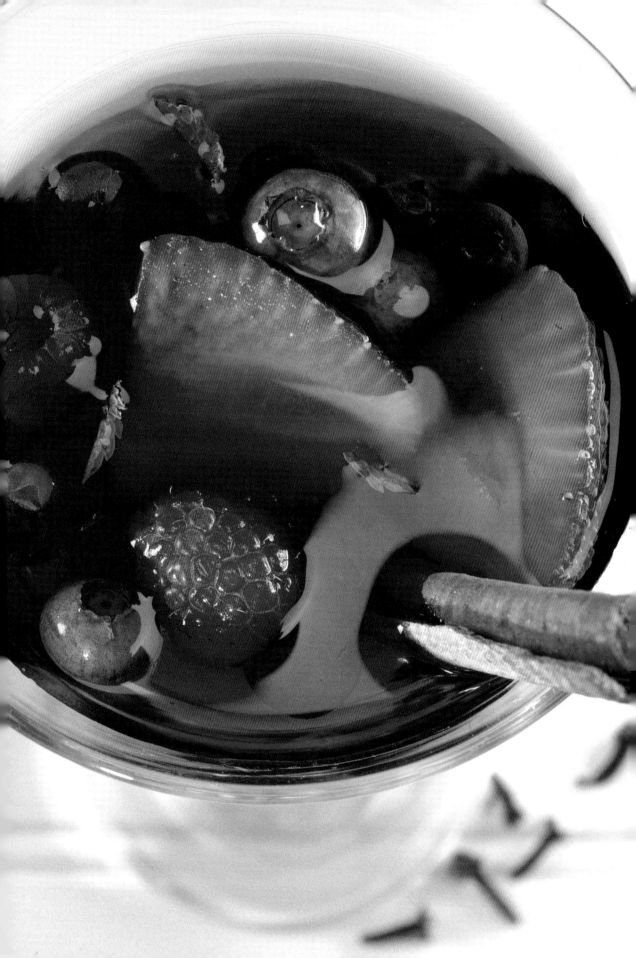

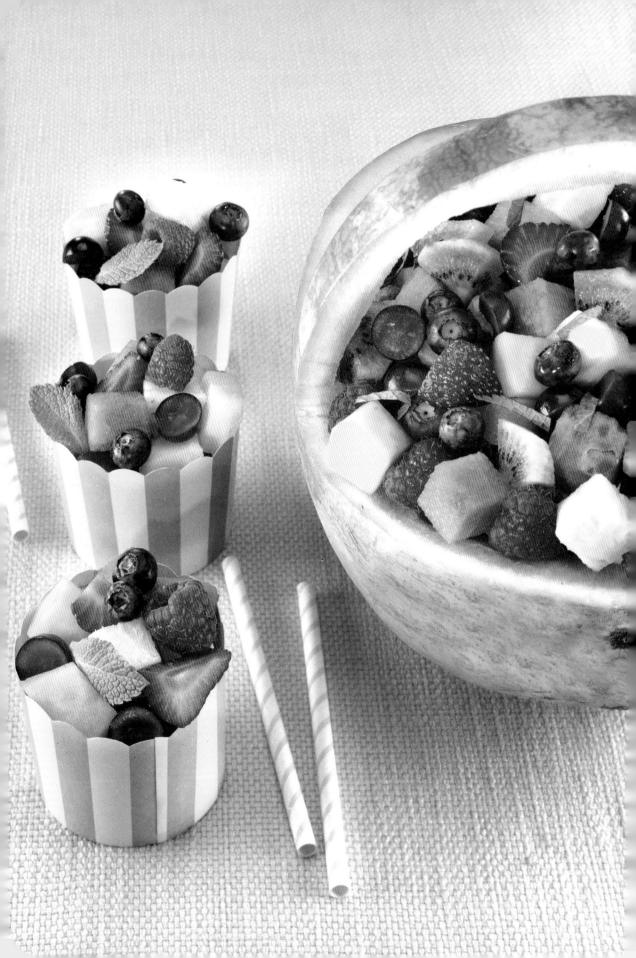

FRESH FRUIT
BASKET

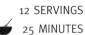

12 SERVINGS

25 MINUTES

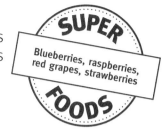

SUPER

Blueberries, raspberries, red grapes, strawberries

FOODS

INGREDIENTS

1 large watermelon, seeded

1 honeydew melon, cubed

1 cup (250 ml) **red grapes**, halved

25 **strawberries**, quartered

3 kiwis, peeled and cubed

1 pineapple, cubed

1 cup (250 ml) **blueberries**

1 cup (250 ml) **raspberries**

2 tbsp chopped fresh mint

METHOD

Carve watermelon into basket with handle.

Remove flesh and cut in cubes.

In a large bowl, combine fruit with mint. Transfer to melon basket.

——— HOW TO SELECT GRAPES ———

Opt for full, plump clusters and make sure the grapes are firmly attached to the stems. Remember to always thoroughly rinse grapes prior to consumption.

Nutrition Facts Per serving	
Amount	% Daily Value
Calories 90	
Fat 0.5 g	1%
Saturated 0.1 g + Trans 0 g	
Polyunsaturated 0.2 g	
Omega-6 0.2 g	
Omega-3 0.1 g	
Monounsaturated 0.1 g	
Cholesterol 0 mg	0%
Sodium 10 mg	0%
Potassium 330 mg	9%
Carbohydrates 21 g	7%
Fiber 3 g	12%
Sugar 15 g	
Protein 1 g	
Vitamin A 156 ER	15%
Vitamin C 66 mg	110%
Calcium 27 mg	2%
Iron 0.6 mg	4%
Phosphorus 31.6 mg	2%

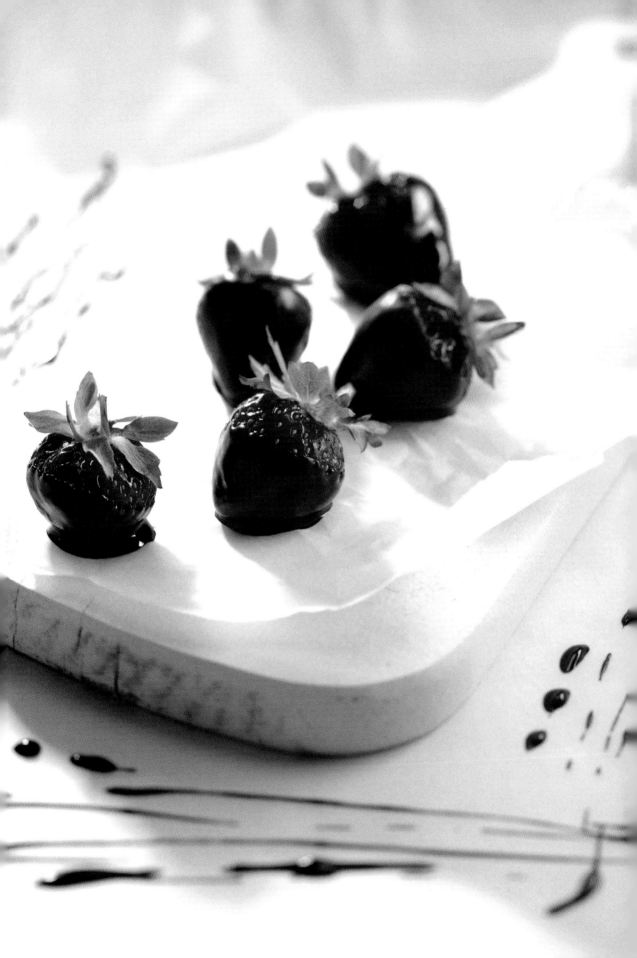

CHOCOLATE
STRAWBERRIES

4 SERVINGS

5 MINUTES

10 MINUTES

❄ 35 MINUTES

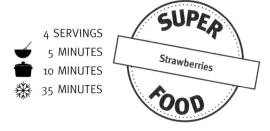

SUPER
Strawberries
FOOD

INGREDIENTS

½ cup (125 ml) dark chocolate (70% cacao or higher)

20 **strawberries**, refrigerated at least 30 minutes

METHOD

In a saucepan or double boiler over low heat, melt chocolate, stirring constantly, for about 5 minutes.

Line a tray or cookie sheet with parchment paper. Dip strawberry ends in chocolate. Place on prepared cookie sheet.

Refrigerate for 5 minutes.

——— CHEF'S TIP ———

Strawberries should be rinsed prior to being hulled to avoid filling with liquid.

Nutrition Facts Per serving	
Amount	**% Daily Value**
Calories 180	
Fat 14 g	22%
Saturated 8 g + Trans 0 g	
Polyunsaturated 0.1 g	
Omega-6 0 g	
Omega-3 0 g	
Monounsaturated 0 g	
Cholesterol 0 mg	0%
Sodium 0 mg	0%
Potassium 55 mg	2%
Carbohydrates 11 g	4%
Fiber 4 g	16%
Sugar 2 g	
Protein 3 g	
Vitamin A 0 ER	0%
Vitamin C 21 mg	35%
Calcium 25 mg	2%
Iron 3.3 mg	25%
Phosphorus 8.4 mg	0%

RAW WALNUT
BARS

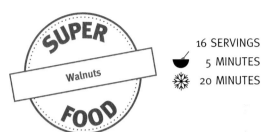

16 SERVINGS
5 MINUTES
20 MINUTES

INGREDIENTS

3 cups (750 ml) **walnuts**

20 dates, pitted

½ cup (125 ml) peanut or almond butter

½ cup (125 ml) cocoa powder

METHOD

Line a 9 x 9 inch (23 x 23 cm) baking pan with parchment paper.

In a food processor, pulse nuts until crumbly. Add remaining ingredients and continue blending until mixture forms a sticky ball. Press mixture into pan using your hands.

Refrigerate for 20 minutes. Cut into bars.

Variation: Following the same procedure, roll mixture into 16 balls instead.

Nutrition Facts Per serving	
Amount	**% Daily Value**
Calories 250	
Fat 18 g	28%
Saturated 2 g	
+ Trans 0 g	
Polyunsaturated 12 g	
Omega-6 9 g	
Omega-3 2 g	
Monounsaturated 3.5 g	
Cholesterol 0 mg	0%
Sodium 15 mg	1%
Potassium 240 mg	7%
Carbohydrates 15 g	5%
Fiber 2 g	8%
Sugar 9 g	
Protein 6 g	
Vitamin A 1 ER	0%
Vitamin C 0 mg	0%
Calcium 30 mg	2%
Iron 0.8 mg	6%
Phosphorus 94.1 mg	8%

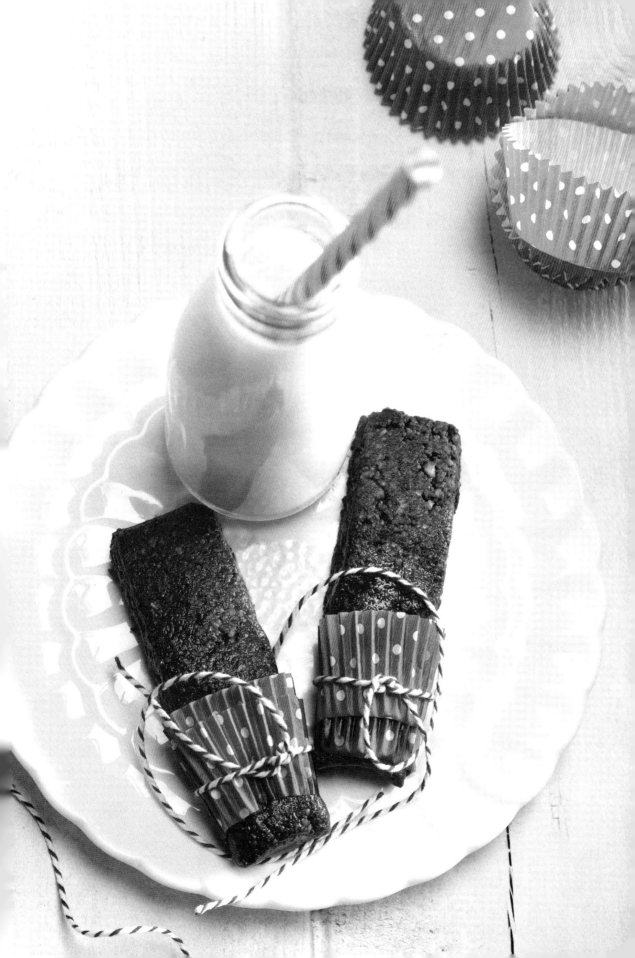

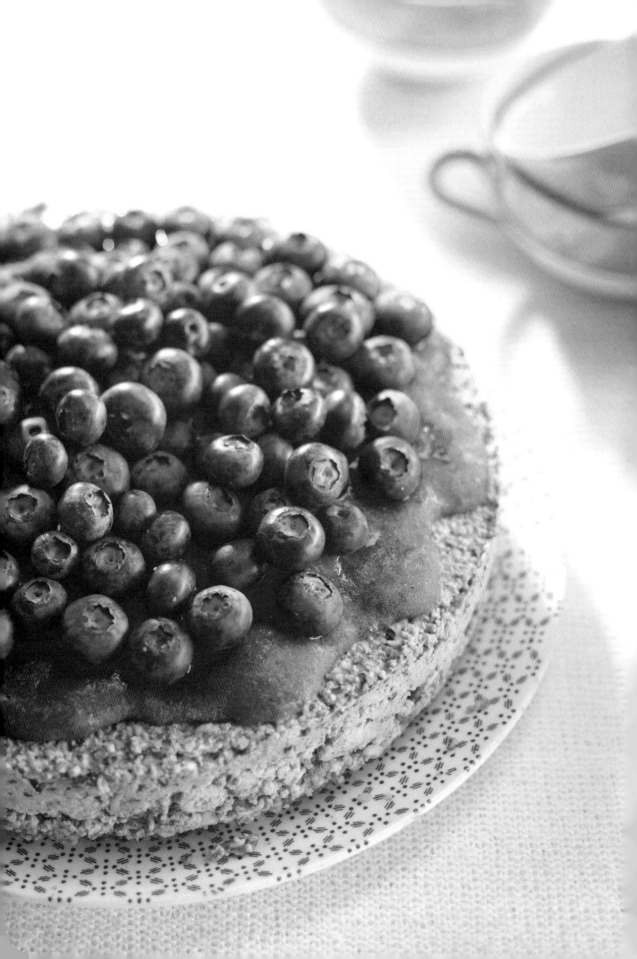

RAW BLUEBERRY, STRAWBERRY
AND NUT PIE

 16 SERVINGS
OVERNIGHT
30 MINUTES
4 TO 5 HOURS
10 MINUTES

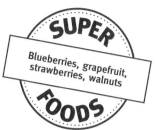
Blueberries, grapefruit, strawberries, walnuts

INGREDIENTS

For the crust

2 tbsp coconut milk

1 tbsp coconut oil

1 cup (250 ml) oat bran

¼ cup (60 ml) pecans

¼ cup (60 ml) almonds

¼ cup (60 ml) **walnuts**

8 dried dates, pitted and chopped

1 tsp vanilla extract

For the topping

2 tbsp coconut oil

1 tsp vanilla extract

2 cups (500 ml) hazelnuts, soaked overnight

1 cup (250 ml) **blueberries**

1 cup (250 ml) **strawberries**

For the purée

2 cups (500 ml) **strawberries**

2 tbsp **grapefruit** juice

For the garnish

2 cups (500 ml) **blueberries**

METHOD

In a food processor, blend all ingredients for the crust at high speed until mixture forms a sticky ball. Add more dates or water, if needed. Press mixture into 9-inch (23 cm) springform pan.

In a food processor, blend all ingredients for the topping. Spread evenly over crust using a spatula.

Cover pie with aluminum foil or plastic wrap. Freeze for 4 to 5 hours.

In a blender, purée strawberries and grapefruit juice. Transfer to a bowl, cover with aluminum foil and refrigerate for 10 minutes.

Spread strawberry purée evenly over pie. Refrigerate or serve immediately. Top pie with blueberries prior to serving.

Nutrition Facts Per serving	
Amount	% Daily Value
Calories 260	
Fat 18 g	28%
Saturated 3 g + Trans 0 g	
Polyunsaturated 2.5 g	
Omega-6 2.5 g	
Omega-3 0.2 g	
Monounsaturated 11 g	
Cholesterol 0 mg	0%
Sodium 25 mg	1%
Potassium 250 mg	7%
Carbohydrates 19 g	6%
Fiber 4 g	16%
Sugar 9 g	
Protein 5 g	
Vitamin A 4 ER	0%
Vitamin C 20 mg	35%
Calcium 55 mg	4%
Iron 1.9 mg	15%
Phosphorus 130.4 mg	10%

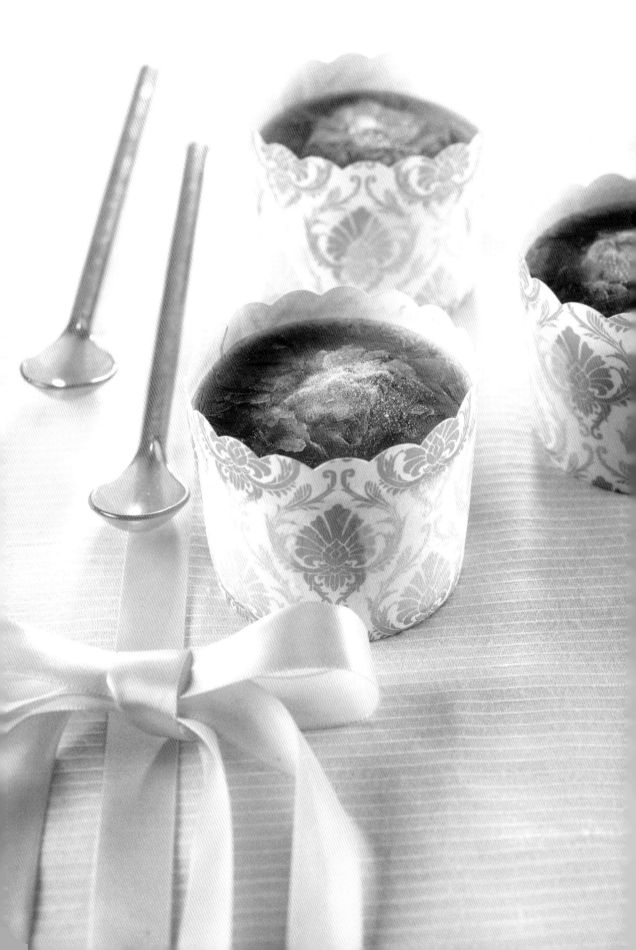

FRUITY FROZEN
YOGURT

4 SERVINGS
15 MINUTES
4 TO 6 HOURS

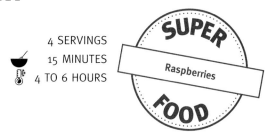

SUPER
Raspberries
FOOD

INGREDIENTS

1 very ripe banana

1 cup (250 ml) fresh **raspberries**

1 cup (250 ml) diced watermelon

1 cup (250 ml) plain Greek 0% M.F. yogurt

METHOD

In a food processor, blend all ingredients until smooth.

Divide mixture into bowls and gently tap bowls against counter to remove air bubbles.

Freeze for 4 to 6 hours or until firm.

Nutrition Facts Per serving	
Amount	**% Daily Value**
Calories 100	
Fat 0.5 g	1%
Saturated 0.2 g	
+ Trans 0 g	
Polyunsaturated 0.2 g	
Omega-6 0.1 g	
Omega-3 0.1 g	
Monounsaturated 0 g	
Cholesterol 1 mg	0%
Sodium 35 mg	2%
Potassium 200 mg	6%
Carbohydrates 16 g	5%
Fiber 3 g	12%
Sugar 9 g	
Protein 8 g	
Vitamin A 26 ER	2%
Vitamin C 14 mg	25%
Calcium 74 mg	6%
Iron 0.4 mg	2%
Phosphorus 20.1 mg	2%

RASPBERRY KIWI
POPS

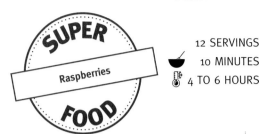

SUPER FOOD
Raspberries

12 SERVINGS
10 MINUTES
4 TO 6 HOURS

INGREDIENTS

2 cups (500 ml) plain Greek 0% M.F. yogurt

Drizzle maple syrup

2 cups (500 ml) fresh or frozen **raspberries**

1 cup (250 ml) thinly sliced kiwis

METHOD

In a blender or food processor, blend all ingredients until smooth.

Divide mixture into Popsicle molds. Gently tap molds against counter to remove air bubbles. Insert a stick in center of each mold.

Freeze for 4 to 6 hours or until firm.

Pass molds under hot water to unstick pops. Serve immediately.

Nutrition Facts Per serving	
Amount	**% Daily Value**
Calories 50	
Fat 0.3 g	0%
Saturated 0 g	
+ Trans 0 g	
Polyunsaturated 0.1 g	
Omega-6 0.1 g	
Omega-3 0 g	
Monounsaturated 0 g	
Cholesterol 1 mg	0%
Sodium 30 mg	1%
Potassium 190 mg	5%
Carbohydrates 9 g	3%
Fiber 2 g	8%
Sugar 7 g	
Protein 3 g	
Vitamin A 3 ER	0%
Vitamin C 21 mg	35%
Calcium 85 mg	8%
Iron 0.3 mg	2%
Phosphorus 70.7 mg	6%

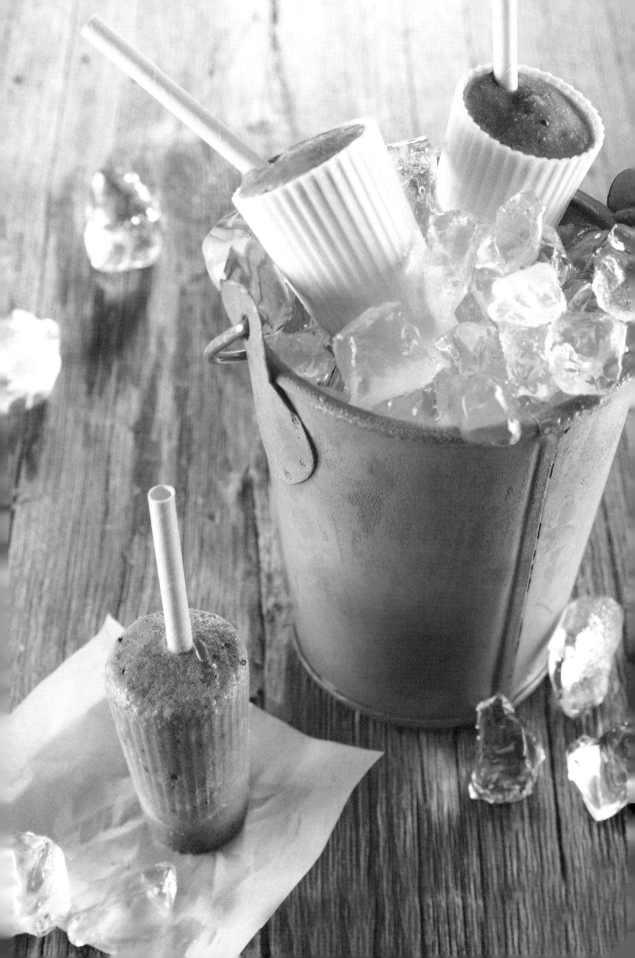

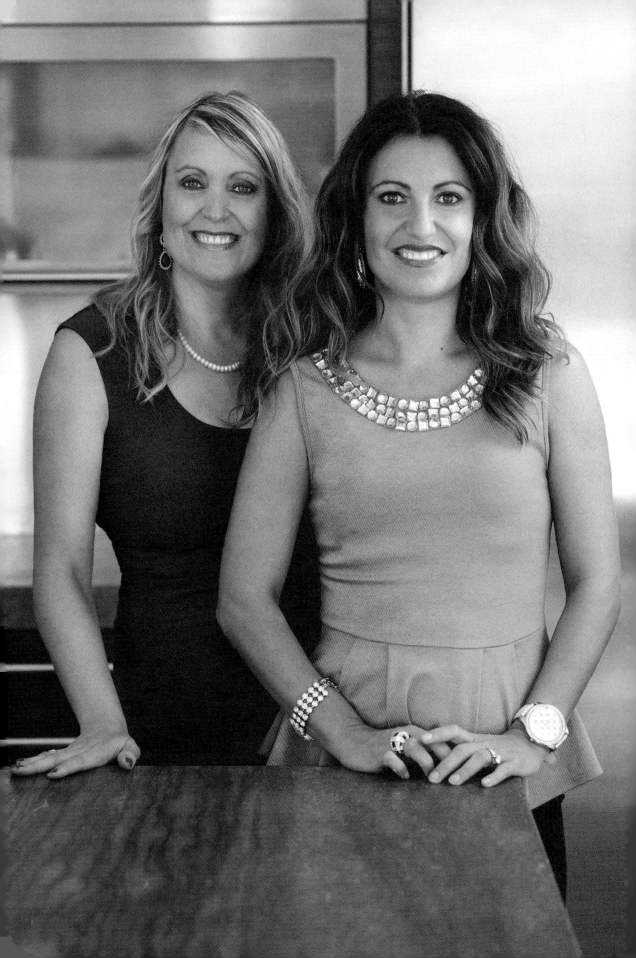

ACKNOWLEDGMENTS

Thank you to Marc G. Alain and Isabelle Jodoin at Modus Vivendi Publishing for giving us the chance to be part of the new Superfoods series. Thanks to Nolwenn Gouezel, who offered invaluable assistance researching and writing this book. Thanks also to Émilie Houle, graphic designer.

Thanks to photographer André Noël and food stylist Gabrielle Dalessandro for making our recipes even more appetizing, as well as Camille Gyrya for our photos and other pictures.

Thank you to our science committee for verifying the information.

Thanks to our chef, Michael Linnington, who added his delicate touch to our recipes.

And thanks to the loves of our lives: our spouses, Jack and Pierre, who patiently supported us while we wrote this book, and our children, Eza, Oceana, Xavier and Jessica, Dominique and Valérie, who drive us to follow our dreams.

We hope with all our hearts that you achieve your life's goals.

Thank you to everyone who buys this book or consults us at a clinic. Be sure to visit our website (nutrisimple.com).

Marise Charron and Elisabeth Cerqueira
nutrisimple.com

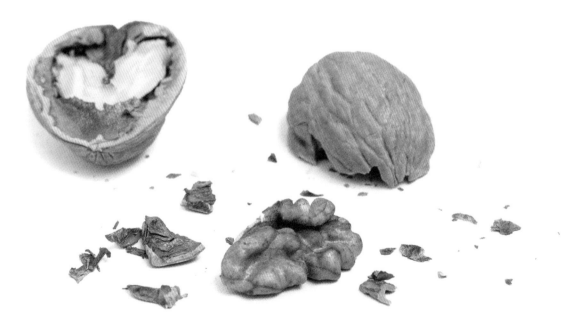

SCIENTIFIC
REFERENCES

Adams, L. S., S. Phung, N. Yee, N. Seeram, L. Li, and S. Chen. "Blueberry phytochemicals inhibit growth and metastatic potential of MDA-MB-231 breast cancer cells through modulation of the phosphatidylinositol 3-kinase pathway." *Cancer Research* 70 (2010): 3594–605.

Aslam, T., C. Delcourt, R. Silva, F. G. Holz, A. Leys, A. Garcia Layana, and E. Souled. "Micronutrients in age-related macular degeneration." *Ophthalmologica* 229, no. 2 (2013): 75–79.

Bae, J. M., E. J. Lee, and G. Guyatt. "Citrus fruit intake and stomach cancer risk: a quantitative systematic review." *Gastric Cancer* 11 (2008): 23–32.

Bazzano, L. A., J. He, L. G. Ogden et al. "Legume consumption and risk of coronary heart disease in US men and women: NHANES I Epidemiologic Follow-up Study." *Archives of Internal Medicine* 161, no. 21 (2001): 2573–78.

Béliveau, R. "Adoptez les poissons gras." Prévention du cancer, *Journal de Montréal*, October 2, 2006. http://www.richardbeliveau.org/images/chroniques/R2006-10-02-OCT-049--CompressedSecured.pdf.

Béliveau, R. "Bien manger pour contrer le déclin cognitif." Accessed June 22, 2013. http://www.cogir.net/DATA/NOUVELLE/82_fr~v~la-chronique-de-richard-beliveau-bien-manger-pour-contrer-le-declin-cognitif.pdf.

Béliveau, R. "Des bleuets pour prévenir le cancer du sein." Prévention, *Journal de Montréal*, August 16, 2010. http://www.richardbeliveau.org/images/chroniques/R2010-08-16-AOU-041--CompressedSecured.pdf.

Béliveau, R. "Des noix à manger sans modération." Prévention, *Journal de Montréal*, December 21, 2009. http://www.richardbeliveau.org/images/chroniques/R2009-12-21-DEC-047--CompressedSecured.pdf.

Béliveau, R. "Faites le plein de petits fruits." Prévention du cancer, *Journal de Montréal*, May 28, 2007. http://www.richardbeliveau.org/images/chroniques/R2007-05-28-MAI-051--CompressedSecured.pdf.

Bertelli, A. A., and D. K. Das. "Grapes, wines, resveratrol and heart health." *Journal of Cardiovascular Pharmacology* 54, no. 6 (2009): 468–76.

Boivin, D., M. Blanchette, S. Barrette, A. Moghrabi, and R. Béliveau. "Inhibition of cancer cell proliferation and suppression of TNF-induced activation of NFkappaB by edible berry juice." *Anticancer Research* 27, no. 2 (2007): 937–48.

Burton-Freeman, B., A. Linares, D. Hyson et al. "Strawberry modulates LDL oxidation and post-prandial lipemia in response to high-fat meal in overweight hyperlipidemic men and women." *The Journal of the American College of Nutrition* 29 no. 1 (2010): 46–54.

Celec, P., D. Ostatnikova, M. Caganova et al. "Endocrine and cognitive effects of short-time soybean consumption in women." *Gynecologic and Obstetric Investigation* 59 (2005): 62–66.

Chainani-Wu, N. "Diet and oral, pharyngeal, and esophageal cancer." *Nutrition and Cancer* 44, no. 2 (2002): 104–26.

Coates, E. M., G. Popa, C. I. R. Gill, M. J. McCann, G. J. McDougall, D. Stewart, and I. Rowland. "Colon-available raspberry polyphenols exhibit anti-cancer effects on in vitro models of colon cancer." *Journal of Carcinogenesis* 6 (2007): 4–17.

Collectif. "Tout sur les fruits, les noix et les graines." In *L'Encyclopédie des aliments*, Vol. 2. Montreal: Québec Amérique, 2014.

Collectif. "Tout sur les légumes." In *L'Encyclopédie des aliments*, Vol. 1. Montreal: Québec Amérique, 2013.

Colquhoun, D. M., D. Moores, S. M. Somerset, and J. A. Humphries. "Comparison of the effects on lipoproteins and apolipoproteins of a diet high in monounsaturated fatty acids, enriched with avocado, and a high-carbohydrate diet." *American Journal of Clinical Nutrition* 56, no. 4 (1992): 671–77.

Cosgrove, M. C., O. H. Franco, S. P. Granger, P. G. Murray, and A. E. Mayes. "Dietary nutrient intakes and skin-aging appearance among middle-aged American women." *American Journal of Clinical Nutrition* 86, no. 4 (2007): 1225–31.

Delaby, M. N. "Santé: les mangeurs de noix vivent plus longtemps." *Le Figaro*. Accessed May 2014. http://sante.lefigaro.fr/actualite/2013/11/29/21589-mangeurs-noix-vivent-plus-longtemps.

Devore, E. E., J. H. Kang, M. M. Breteler, and F. Grodstein. "Dietary intakes of berries and flavonoids in relation to cognitive decline." *Annuals of Neurology* 72 (2012): 135–43.

Fleischauer, A. T., C. Poole, and L. Arab. "Garlic consumption and cancer prevention: meta-analyses of colorectal and stomach cancers." *American Journal of Clinical Nutrition* 72, no. 4 (2000): 1047–52.

Folts, J. D. "Potential health benefits from the flavonoids in grape products on vascular disease." *Advances in Experimental Medicine and Biology* 505 (2002): 95–111.

Foschi, R., C. Pelucchi, M. L. Dal et al. "Citrus fruit and cancer risk in a network of case-control studies." *Cancer Causes & Control* 21 (2010): 237–42.

Galeone, C., C. Pelucchi, F. Levi et al. "Onion and garlic use and human cancer." *American Journal of Clinical Nutrition* 84, no. 5 (2006): 1027–32.

Gorinstein, S., A. Caspi et al. "Preventive effects of diets supplemented with sweetie fruits in hypercholesterolemic patients suffering from coronary artery disease." *Preventive Medicine* 38, no. 6 (2004): 841–47.

Hannum, S. M. "Potential impact of strawberries on human health: a review of the science." *Critical Reviews in Food Science and Nutrition* 44, no. 1 (2004): 1–17.

Heinonen, I. M., A. S. Meyer, and A. N. Frankel. "Antioxidant activity of berry phenolics on human low-density lipoprotein and liposome oxidation." *Journal of Agricultural and Food Chemistry* 46 (1998): 4107–12.

Jenab, M., P. Ferrari et al. "Association of nut and seed intake with colorectal cancer risk in the European Prospective Investigation into Cancer and Nutrition." *Cancer Epidemiology, Biomarkers & Prevention* 13, no. 10 (2004): 1595–603.

Jian, L., A. H. Lee, and C. W. Binns. "Tea and lycopene protect against prostate cancer." *Asia Pacific Journal of Clinical Nutrition* 16, suppl. 1 (2007): 453–57.

Joseph, J. A., B. Shukitt-Hale, and G. Casadesus. "Reversing the deleterious effects of aging on neuronal communication and behavior: beneficial properties of fruit polyphenolic compounds." *American Journal of Clinical Nutrition* 81, suppl. 1 (2005): 313S–316S.

Kirsh, V. A., U. Peters, S. T. Mayne et al. "Prospective study of fruit and vegetable intake and risk of prostate cancer." *Journal of the National Cancer Institute* 99 (2007): 1200–9.

Krikorian, R., T. A. Nash et al. "Concord grape juice supplementation improves memory function in older adults with mild cognitive impairment." *British Journal of Nutrition* 103 (2010): 730–34.

Lanza, E., T. J. Hartman, P. S. Albert et al. "High dry bean intake and reduced risk of advanced colorectal adenoma recurrence among participants in the polyp prevention trial." *Journal of Nutrition* 136, no. 7 (2006): 1896–903.

Lin, J., K. M. Rexrode, F. Hu et al. "Dietary intakes of flavonols and flavones and coronary heart disease in US women." *American Journal of Epidemiology* 165 (2007): 1305–13.

Lu, Q. Y., J. R. Arteaga, Q. Zhang, S. Huerta, V. L. W. Go, and D. Heber. "Inhibition of prostate cancer cell growth by an avocado extract: role of lipid-soluble bioactive substances." *Journal of Nutritional Biochemistry* 16 (2005): 23–30.

Mukuddem-Petersen, J., W. Oosthuizen, and J. C. Jerling. "A systematic review of the effects of nuts on blood lipid profiles in humans." *Journal of Nutrition* 135, no. 9 (2005): 2082–89.

National Eye Institute. "What the age-related eye disease studies mean for you." Accessed May 2014. https://www.nei.nih.gov/areds2/PatientFAQ.

Naulleau, C. "Les noix et leurs vertus." Espaces, November 2008. Accessed September 13, 2013. http://www.espaces.ca/categorie/conseils/nutrition/article/481-les-noix-et-leurs-vertus.

Pan, S. Y., A. M. Ugnat, Y. Mao, S. W. Wen, and K. C. Johnson. "A case-control study of diet and the risk of ovarian cancer." *Cancer Epidemiology, Biomarkers & Prevention* 13, no. 9 (2004): 1521–27.

Passeportsante.net. "Noix." Accessed September 13, 2013. http://www.passeportsante.net/fr/Nutrition/EncyclopedieAliments/Fiche.aspx?doc=noix_nu.

Pattison, D., A. Silman, N. Goodson et al. "Vitamin C and the risk of developing inflammatory polyarthritis: prospective nested case-control study." *Annals of the Rheumatic Disease* 63, no. 7 (2004): 843–47.

Ribaya-Mercado, J. D., and J. B. Blumberg. "Lutein and zeaxanthin and their potential roles in disease prevention." *American Journal of Clinical Nutrition* 23, suppl. 6 (2004): 567S–587S.

Tamimi, R. M., S. E. Hankinson, H. Campos et al. "Plasma carotenoids, retinol, and tocopherols and risk of breast cancer." *American Journal of Epidemiology* 161, no. 2 (2005): 153–60.

Van Leeuwen, R., S. Boekhoorn, J. R. Vingerling et al. "Dietary intake of antioxidants and risk of age-related macular degeneration." *Journal of the American Medical Association* 294, no. 24 (2005): 3101–7.

Yuan, J. M., D. O. Stram, K. Arakawa, H. P. Lee, and M. C. Yu. "Dietary cryptoxanthin and reduced risk of lung cancer: the Singapore Chinese Health Study." *Cancer Epidemiology, Biomarkers & Prevention* 12, no. 9 (2003): 890–98.

Zamora-Ros, R., M. Rabassa, A. Cherubini, M. Urpi-Sardà, S. Bandinelli, L. Ferrucci, and C. Andres-Lacueva. "High concentrations of a urinary biomarker of polyphenol intake are associated with decreased mortality in older adults." *Journal of Nutrition* 143, no. 9 (2013): 1445–50.

Zhang, X., X. O. Shu, Y. B. Xiang et al. "Cruciferous vegetable consumption is associated with a reduced risk of total and cardiovascular disease mortality." *American Journal of Clinical Nutrition* 94 (2011): 240–46.

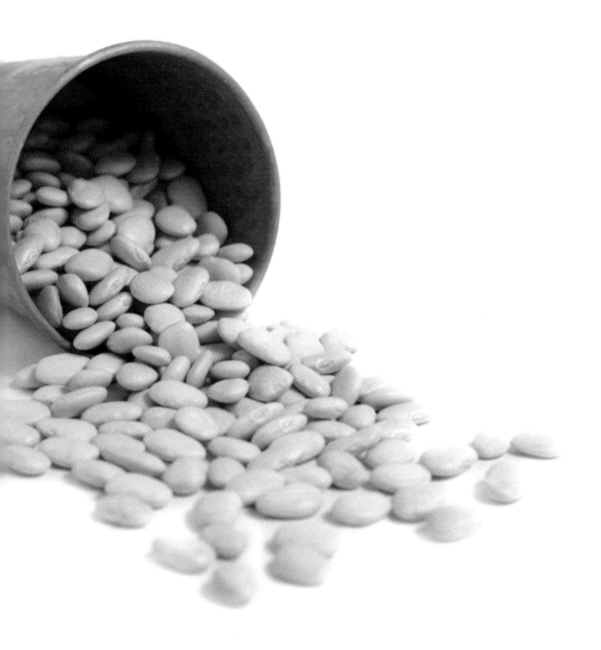

GLOSSARY

ALLICIN
Chemical substance that forms when garlic is crushed or minced. Responsible for garlic's strong aroma, allicin produces several sulfur compounds beneficial to our health. To help produce allicin and benefit from its virtues, it is recommended to crush garlic and let it sit 10 minutes prior to cooking with it. In order to preserve its heat-sensitive nutrients, garlic should be added to dishes only during the last 20 minutes of cooking.

AMINO ACIDS
Elements that make up proteins. The body needs 20 amino acids to grow and function, but it produces only 11 of them. The nine others are called essential, because the human body cannot produce them so they have to come exclusively from diet. *See* Protein.

ANTHOCYANIN
Pigments that give certain blue and red fruits and vegetables their color (blueberries, blackcurrants, cranberries, cherries, etc.). They belong to the flavonoid family.

ANTIOXIDANTS
Compounds that help prevent oxidative stress caused by free radicals. Vitamins C and E, selenium, carotenoids and polyphenols are among the most antioxidant substances.

BETA-CAROTENE
Carotene precursor of vitamin A. This powerful antioxidant is found mainly in yellow, orange and red fruits and vegetables (for example, carrots, pumpkins and sweet potatoes) as well as in leafy green vegetables (such as spinach and Brussels sprouts), where the pigment is masked by the chlorophyll.

CALCIUM
Mineral essential to the formation and development of bones and teeth. Not only does calcium strengthen bones, it also plays an important role in healing wounds and muscle contraction and relaxation. It is involved in regulating blood pressure, normalizing the heartbeat and transmitting messages from the nervous system. The best sources of calcium are dairy products and substitutes. Canned fished (such as sardines and salmon) are also good sources if the bones are eaten. Leafy green vegetables, such as broccoli and cabbage, also provide calcium, but in lesser amounts. Calcium from legumes, nuts and seeds is not as easily absorbed by the body as calcium from dairy products.

CARBOHYDRATES

The body's main source of energy. The complex carbohydrates contained, for example, in whole-grain products, vegetables, fruits and legumes are best. A diet with complex carbohydrates can protect against heart disease and stabilize blood sugar.

CAROTENOIDS

Pigments that give fruits and vegetables a yellow, orange or red color. Carotenoids are powerful antioxidants that act preventatively against certain degenerative illnesses. They protect cells exposed to ultraviolet rays from oxidative damage. According to a number of studies, they may slow the growth of cancerous tumors. Carotenoids include lutein and zeaxanthin, lycopene (found in tomatoes), capsanthin (found in red peppers) and beta-carotene, a precursor to vitamin A.

CHOLINE

A B complex vitamin component. Choline promotes proper brain functioning and improves memory; it may slow the progression of Alzheimer's disease and dementia. It is found mainly in egg yolk, but also in liver, meat, fish, peanuts and nuts.

COLLAGEN

Fibrous protein in the body that acts as the main component of connective tissue.

COPPER

A trace element that helps fight against free radicals. Copper also helps in the formation of red blood cells and many hormones. It is found in mollusks and shellfish, meat, nuts, seeds and legumes.

ESSENTIAL FATTY ACIDS

Polyunsaturated fats called essential because the body cannot make them, and they are needed for its functioning and development. *See* Omega-3s.

FIBER

Carbohydrates that the body cannot digest. Fiber arrives intact in the large intestine, where it ferments under the effects of intestinal bacteria. The health benefits of fiber come from this fermentation. It is found in foods of plant origin (foods of animal origin contain virtually no fiber). There are two major families of fiber: soluble fiber and insoluble fiber.

FLAVONOIDS

Phytochemical compounds in the family of polyphenols. Whether isoflavonoids, quercetin, anthocyanins, anthocyanidines, flavonols or flavones, all of these compounds appear to limit oxidative damage caused by free radicals. In addition to reducing inflammation that can lead to atherosclerosis, therefore to heart disease, they can play a role in preventing cancer. Flavonoids are found in colorful fruits and vegetables.

FOLATE

Vitamin B_9, more commonly known as folic acid, is the synthetic form of folate. *See* Vitamin B complex.

FREE RADICALS

Molecules naturally produced by the body through breathing and the digestion of food. While they help the body get rid of certain viruses, germs and bacteria, even its own cells when they are damaged, free radicals become harmful when too many of them are produced. They damage cells and limit their ability to regenerate. This excess of free radicals is called oxidative stress. Our body has an internal antioxidant system that gets rid of free radicals but antioxidants in diet may be of valuable help.

HEME IRON

Type of iron found in animal products. Heme iron (also called haem iron) is the best source of iron for the body, because it is easier to assimilate than plant-based iron.

INSOLUBLE FIBER

Fiber that helps regulate intestinal transit and creates a feeling of fullness. It is found primarily in the peel of fruits and vegetables, whole grains and wheat bran.

IRON

Trace element essential not only to carrying oxygen and the formation of red blood cells, but also to chemical reactions within cells. To better absorb iron, it is a good idea to eat foods rich in vitamin C (e.g., citrus, berries and certain vegetables, such as peppers) in a single meal. There are two types of dietary iron: heme iron and non-heme iron.

LIMONOIDS

Phytochemicals that are part of the terpene family. Limonoids are responsible for giving citrus fruit their distinctive smell. Their antioxidant properties have been shown to prevent cancerous cells from spreading and lower blood cholesterol levels.

LIPIDS

Saturated, polyunsaturated and monounsaturated fatty acids. Lipids provide the body energy and are building blocks for all of the body's cells. They ensure proper brain function and facilitate the absorption of vitamins A, D, E and K. *See* Essential fatty acids, Saturated fatty acids, Unsaturated fatty acids.

LUTEIN AND ZEAXANTHIN

Carotenoid pigments that give vegetables their bright color (yellow, orange, red or green). Abundant in food, lutein and zeaxanthin are essential to good eye health. A diet rich in lutein and zeaxanthin appears to prevent cataracts. The best sources of lutein are leafy green vegetables (e.g., spinach, kale) and eggs. The best sources of zeaxanthin are leafy green vegetables and red pepper.

LYCOPENE

Pigment that gives vegetables a red color. It is the most abundant carotenoid in the human body. Lycopene is a very active antioxidant. It may reduce the risk of prostate cancer and slow its development, and may protect the skin against the free radicals produced by ultraviolet rays. In turn, it also potentially slows skin aging. The best sources are tomatoes and derivatives (e.g., tomato sauce, tomato paste), watermelon, pink or red grapefruit and red pepper.

MAGNESIUM

Mineral that activates over 300 biochemical reactions in the body. Magnesium helps build bones and teeth. It makes muscles and nerves work and maintains a regular heartbeat. Every cell in the body requires magnesium. It is found in green vegetables, legumes, nuts and seeds, cocoa and certain whole-grain products (such as whole wheat bread).

MANGANESE

A trace element that plays an indirect role in a number of metabolic processes and that prevents the damage caused by free radicals. Manganese helps metabolize carbohydrates and fats, in the formation of cartilage and healthy bones and in regulating blood sugar. The best sources are whole grains, nuts and seeds, legumes and certain fruits and vegetables.

MINERALS

Micronutrients that are indispensable to the proper functioning of the body. These include calcium, magnesium, phosphorus, potassium and sodium.

MOLYBDENUM

Trace element that helps with the absorption of iron and plays an important role in bone and teeth development. Molybdenum is found mainly in wheat germ, buckwheat, legumes, dark green vegetables and nuts.

NON-HEME IRON

Type of iron found in plant-based products. The amount of non-heme iron a food delivers depends on the other products consumed in the same meal: for example, meat proteins and vitamin C increase the absorption of non-heme iron from grains, legumes and vegetables. Wine, tea and coffee reduce its absorption.

NUTRIENTS

Substances needed for the body's functioning.

OMEGA-3S

Polyunsaturated fatty acids called essential found in fish and some plants. Fatty fish (e.g., salmon, rainbow trout, mackerel, herring, halibut, tuna, sardines), ground flaxseed and walnuts are good sources of it. It is important to differentiate the three types of omega-3s: alpha-linolenic acid (ALA), mainly from plant sources, eicosapentaenoic acid (EPA) and docosahexaenoic fatty acid (DHA), mainly from marine sources. All of them are beneficial for the body. However, the effects on heart health have been observed particularly with a high intake of omega-3s from fish and fish oil (EPA and DHA). It is a good idea to make it part of your diet two or three times a week. As for omega-3s of plant origin, even though they are not as easy for the body to assimilate, they should be included in your diet.

OXIDATIVE STRESS

An attack that damages the body's cells caused by free radicals. The compounds that fight oxidative stress are called antioxidants. Oxidative stress could be at the source of a number of diseases, including heart disease and cancer.

PHENOLIC ACIDS

Organic compounds that boast antioxidant properties. Ferulic acid, caffeic acid, coumaric acid, ellagic acid and gallic acid are all examples of phenolic acids. Phenolic acids help prevent age-related diseases by neutralizing free radicals.

PHOSPHORUS

One of the most important minerals in the body after calcium. Phosphorus is essential to almost all chemical reactions in the cells. It helps maintain bone and tooth health and produces the energy the body needs. Foods high in protein (meat, poultry, fish, dairy products, eggs, legumes, nuts and seeds) and whole grains are the main sources of it. However, the phosphorus contained in food of plant origin (such as grains, legumes and nuts) is less bioavailable than that contained in food of animal origin.

PHYTONUTRIENTS

Substance of plant origin with nutritional value. These are not vitamins or minerals, but pigments or biologically active compounds. Known for their antioxidant properties, phytonutrients may offer protection against premature aging, cardiovascular disease and cancer. They are sulfur compounds, phytosterols, polyphenols (e.g., flavonoids, phenolic acids, tannins), resveratrol and terpenes (e.g., carotenoids, lutein, zeaxanthin, lycopene).

PHYTOSTEROLS

Phytonutrients that lower LDL cholesterol ("bad" cholesterol), preventing heart disease. According to studies, phytosterols may also have anti-cancer properties. They are found in sesame and sunflower seeds, sesame oil and nuts.

POLYPHENOLS

Antioxidants of plant origin. The family of polyphenols, or phenolic compounds, includes a number of phytonutrients such as flavonoids, phenolic acids and tannins.

POTASSIUM

Mineral necessary for muscle contraction, the contraction and dilatation of blood vessels, and the transmission of nerve impulses. It works closely with sodium and is involved in many biochemical reactions in the body. It also contributes to kidney health and, working with sodium, ensures the body's cells are hydrated. The main sources of potassium are fruits and fresh vegetables, but dairy products and legumes also have it.

PROTEIN

Nutrient present in all of the body's cells, including skin, muscles, hair and blood. Protein is indispensable to the functioning of the heart, contributes to tissue growth and repair, participates in the production of antibodies, hormones, neurotransmitters and enzymes involved in many biochemical reactions. Diet must deliver enough protein for the body, which is unable to build up reserves. Food proteins are amino acid chains that are taken apart by the body then rebuilt to form new proteins that perform different functions. During digestion, proteins divide into smaller molecules called amino acids. There are 20 different amino acids and some are considered essential because the body cannot make them. They come exclusively from diet. Complete proteins, i.e., those that contain all the amino acids essential to the proper functioning of the body, are found in products of animal origin (e.g.: meat, fish, eggs and dairy products). Plants (legumes, nuts and seeds) are also good sources of protein, but they are incomplete. Grains also contain incomplete proteins.

QUERCETIN

Particularly antioxidant phytonutrient. Quercetin offers not only protection against cancer but also provides cardiovascular protection. It is also found in onions, berries, dark chocolate and tea.

RESVERATROL

Phytonutrient that is particularly abundant in the skin of red grapes. Resveratrol is a good ally in fighting aging and cancer because it reverses skin damage related to ultraviolet rays. As an antioxidant, it blocks the action of free radicals in the skin. Red grapes and red wine are two primary sources of resveratrol in the diet.

SATURATED FATTY ACIDS
Fatty acids that are normally solid at room temperature. These include foods of animal origin (meat, lard, dairy products), palm and coconut oils and hydrogenated margarine. Some saturated fatty acids are responsible for increased LDL cholesterol ("bad" cholesterol) in the blood.

SELENIUM
Trace element with very high antioxidant capacity. Selenium protects cells against free radicals. It is also involved in the proper functioning of the immune system, allows for the synthesis of testosterone and fosters the production of healthy sperm. Selenium enters the food chain through plants, which draw the mineral from the soil. The amount of selenium in plants depends on where they are grown. Brazil nuts and seafood are good sources of selenium.

SODIUM
Micronutrient that plays a major role in hydrating the body by controlling, along with potassium, water entering and leaving cells. Sodium is essential to the transmission of nerve impulses and enables muscle contraction. While it is indispensable, it should be consumed in moderation. A proper balance is required. Any excess could contribute to an increase in blood pressure, a risk factor for heart disease, and promote the loss of bone mass. Too little sodium can cause undesirable effects (dehydration, nausea, muscle cramps and vertigo). The main sources of sodium are table salt, fish (canned, marinated or smoked), soy sauce, feta cheese, store-bought foods (e.g., canned soup, deli meat), and dehydrated, dried and smoked foods.

SOLUBLE FIBER
Fiber that slows digestion and the assimilation of food. It lowers blood cholesterol and stabilizes blood sugar. It is found in legumes, nuts, fruits and oat bran.

SULFUR COMPOUNDS
Chemical substance often associated with a strong odor. The name of these substances comes from the fact that there are one or more sulfur atoms in their chemical structure. They are found in cabbage, garlic and onion.

TANNINS
Phytonutrients present in certain plants. Tannins protect plants from parasites. These antioxidant substances give food a bitter taste. Tea and red wine are good sources.

TERPENES
Phytonutrients that include carotenoids, lutein, zeaxanthin, lycopene, beta-carotene and limonoids.

TRACE ELEMENTS

Micronutrients present in very small quantities in the body, but indispensable to its proper functioning. They include copper, iron, manganese, molybdenum, selenium and zinc.

TRANS FATTY ACIDS

Polyunsaturated fatty acids naturally present in milk and the meat of ruminants, but that are mostly made artificially through hydrogenation (an industrial process that transforms liquid oil into solid fat). Industrial trans fatty acids raise LDL cholesterol ("bad" cholesterol) in the blood and reduce the level of HDL cholesterol ("good" cholesterol). They are found in shortening, hydrogenated margarine, store-bought cookies and desserts, industrial bakery products, chips, frying oil and frozen french fries.

UNSATURATED FATTY ACIDS

Monounsaturated and polyunsaturated fatty acids that can help reduce blood cholesterol. They are found in oils, nuts and seeds.

VITAMIN A

Vitamin that contributes to good vision, particularly at night. Vitamin A promotes the growth of bones and tissue that cover different parts of the body (cornea, bronchial tubes, intestine, genital mucus and skin) and strengthens the immune system. The main sources of vitamin A are products of animal origin, including butter, whole milk, cheese and eggs.

VITAMIN B COMPLEX

Group of vitamins that include B_1 (thiamine), B_2 (riboflavin), B_3 (niacin), B_5 (pantothenic acid), B_6, B_9 (*see also* Folate) and B_{12}. These vitamins protect nerve cells and contribute to proper brain functioning. In the body, they work together to promote the proper use of nutrients, help liberate energy and reinforce the immune system.

VITAMIN C

Vitamin that is particularly antioxidizing. Vitamin C is known to strengthen the immune system, but it also stimulates the production of collagen, promotes skin elasticity, accelerates scarring, helps repair damaged tissue and enables the absorption of iron in foods. Vitamin C is found mainly in citrus fruit (e.g., orange, lemon and grapefruit), berries and vegetables (e.g., broccoli, kale and red pepper).

VITAMIN D

Vitamin that is essential for fighting osteoporosis. Vitamin D enables the absorption of calcium and attachment to bones. Calcium and vitamin D work together for bone and tooth health. Present in certain foods, it can also be produced by the body through exposure to the ultraviolet rays of the sun. The best dietary sources of vitamin D are fish (e.g., salmon, sardines), cod liver and cod liver oil, egg yolk, cow's milk, enriched yogurt, enriched orange juice, soy milk and enriched almonds.

VITAMIN E

Vitamin with antioxidant properties. Vitamin E protects cells against the effects of free radicals, which are responsible for the damage caused to cells, contributing to the development of heart disease and cancer. Vitamin E is found in almonds, sunflower seeds, nuts, avocado, vegetable oils (e.g., olive, canola and sunflower), wheat germ and certain dark green leafy vegetables (e.g., spinach, Swiss chard).

VITAMIN K

Vitamin that plays an important role in blood clotting. Its name comes from the Danish koagulation. Promoting the formation of bones, vitamin K prevents osteoporosis. It also plays an important role in cognitive function and promotes nerve impulses. The main sources are green vegetables, vegetable oil and soy derivatives (tofu and edamame).

VITAMINS

Essential nutrients found in trace amounts in the body. Vitamins are essential to chemical reactions that shape our physical and mental health.

ZEAXANTHIN

See Lutein and zeaxanthin.

ZINC

Mineral essential to life. Present in almost all cells, zinc is involved in over 100 different enzymatic reactions. It helps the body fight infection, promotes the healing of injuries and wounds and helps maintain taste and smell. It also enables the normal growth of the fetus during pregnancy, as well as growth of children and teens. Zinc is present in many foods: red meat, poultry, legumes, nuts, seafood (particularly oysters), whole grains and dairy products. However, zinc from animal sources is better absorbed than zinc from grains, legumes and vegetables.

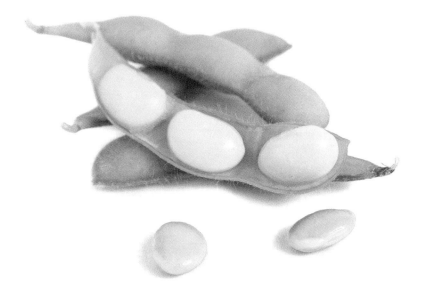

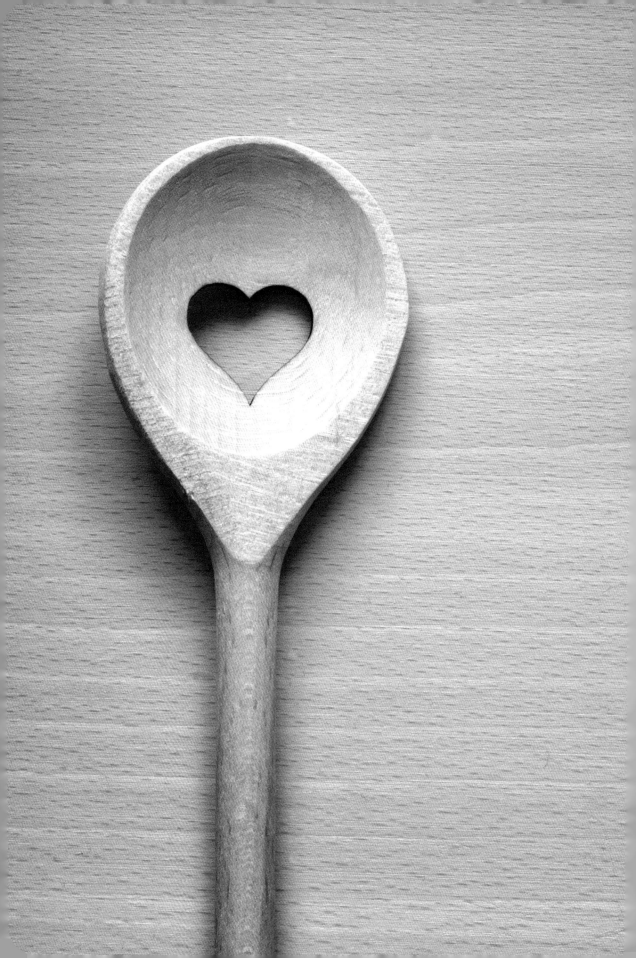

SUPERFOOD
INDEX

AVOCADO

BLUEBERRIES

BROCCOLI

BRUSSELS SPROUTS

EDAMAME

EGGS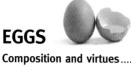

GARLIC

KALE

LIMA BEANS

PINK GRAPEFRUIT

RASPBERRIES

RED GRAPES

RED ONIONS

RED PEPPER

RED WINE

SALMON

SARDINES

STRAWBERRIES

TOMATO

WALNUTS

FROM THE SAME
AUTHORS

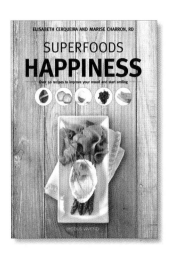

SUPERFOODS HAPPINESS

Low morale, irritability, flagging energy, insomnia . . . Don't wait to do something about it. Find out how your diet can influence your mood and reduce symptoms of depression.

This book features 20 superfoods to lift your mood and over 50 recipes using these fabulous foods: Banana and Green Tea Smoothie, Asparagus Soup, Niçoise Salad with Sardines and Spinach, Beet Chips, Salmon Loaf with Vegetables and Herbs, Portuguese Clams, Lentil and Walnut Balls, Baked Sweet Potato Fries, Chocolaty Mint Dessert, Bakeless Brazil Nut Cake and more.

Superfoods Happiness: everything you need to know to improve your mood and start smiling.

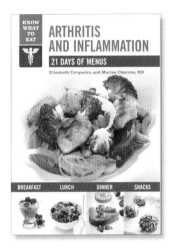

ARTHITIS AND INFLAMMATION

Are your joints swollen and painful? Do you have a hard time getting up in the morning or going up and down stairs? No diet can cure arthritis, but an anti-inflammatory diet can help reduce joint pain.

This guide is specifically designed to help you identifying the best foods for your condition.

Discover delicious recipes that are quick and easy to prepare: Incredible Green Smoothies, Root Vegetable Pâté, Gingery Sweet Potato Soup, Fennel and Orange Salad, Spring Rolls, Kale Stuffed with Poultry and Basmati Rice, Nut-Crusted Salmon, Healthy Truffles, Summer Fruit Salad with Chia Seed and more.

To meet the needs of an even larger audience, the recipes in this book are gluten free.

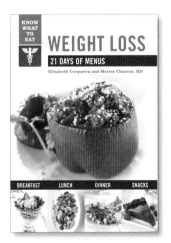

WEIGHT LOSS

Lose weight without drastic dieting, forbidden foods, health risks and, best of all, without regaining the weight you've lost! By changing your lifestyle and adopting healthy eating habits you will be able to manage your weight while enjoying the pleasures of life.

This guide is specifically designed to help you fulfill your nutritional needs without feeling hungry.

Discover recipes that are tasty, simple and quick to prepare: Chicken Quesadillas, Brussels Sprout Chips, Quiche in Quinoa Crust, Marinated Salmon with Mango Salsa, Zucchini Lasagna with Seafood, Portuguese-Style Roast Chicken, Almond-Chocolate Shortcrust Pie, Date Tiramisu and more.

MODUSVIVENDIPUBLISHING.COM